OLGA MOROZOVA

Tick-borne encephalitis vaccines: past, present, and future

AF209882

OLGA MOROZOVA

Tick-borne encephalitis vaccines: past, present, and future

Formalin-inactivated vaccines, DNA and RNA vaccines, recombinant bacteria, multiple antigenic peptides from B- and T-cell epitopes.

ScienciaScripts

Imprint

Any brand names and product names mentioned in this book are subject to trademark, brand or patent protection and are trademarks or registered trademarks of their respective holders. The use of brand names, product names, common names, trade names, product descriptions etc. even without a particular marking in this work is in no way to be construed to mean that such names may be regarded as unrestricted in respect of trademark and brand protection legislation and could thus be used by anyone.

Cover image: www.ingimage.com

This book is a translation from the original published under ISBN 978-3-8433-1159-5.

Publisher:
Sciencia Scripts
is a trademark of
Dodo Books Indian Ocean Ltd. and OmniScriptum S.R.L publishing group

120 High Road, East Finchley, London, N2 9ED, United Kingdom
Str. Armeneasca 28/1, office 1, Chisinau MD-2012, Republic of Moldova, Europe
Managing Directors: Ieva Konstantinova, Victoria Ursu
info@omniscriptum.com

Printed at: see last page
ISBN: 978-620-3-33747-1

Contents

Introduction

For specific prophylaxis of flavivirus infections, inactivated vaccines are currently used predominantly worldwide, with the exception of live attenuated vaccines against yellow fever and Japanese encephalitis viruses. Six types of tick-borne encephalitis vaccines obtained by formalin inactivation of tick-borne encephalitis virus (BTV) from primary cultures of chicken embryonic fibroblasts are currently approved in Russia. Domestically produced inactivated vaccines are based on Far Eastern VEE strains and foreign produced vaccines are based on European strains, which does not match the dominant VEE variants of the Siberian genetic type in most endemic areas of Russia and neighboring countries. Coverage of the population of endemic areas of Russia by vaccination against tick-borne encephalitis varies on average from 5 to 7%, so it has no significant effect on the periodically changing levels of morbidity of the endemic areas population with tick-borne encephalitis. The long-term scheme of three-times immunization and the need for revaccination every three years necessitates the search for new ways to prevent not only tick-borne encephalitis, but also other flavivirus infections ecologically associated with ticks.

In the 1990s, after determining the primary structures of the full-length genomes of vaccine strains of VEE, the E, M, and NS1 genes on the surface of virions and infected cells, respectively, were cloned into eukaryotic expression vectors. Vaccination of laboratory mice with recombinant plasmid DNA with cloned prM, E, and NS1 VCE genes under the control of promoters recognized by eukaryotic RNA polymerases revealed a protective effect of DNA immunization only against a homologous strain of the virus in the absence of viral neutralizing antibodies. Injections of the plasmid with the VKE NS3 gene did not provide a protective effect. The recombinant plasmid DNA was unstable in eukaryotic cells. At 10 h after intramuscular injection, 0.001% remained, and at 24 h 0.0000001% of the original plasmid. In addition, genetic rearrangements of recombinant plasmids and integration into cell chromosomes were detected. Gene immunization with recombinant RNA excludes the possibility of chromosomal rearrangements in host cells, but RNA cleavage requires repeated injections. For recombinant RNAs, a protective effect was found only after administration of full-length genomic RNAs, but not genome fragments containing E and NS1 surface antigen genes. Construction of recombinant and chimeric flaviviruses does not ensure homogeneity of genomic RNA of viral quasispecies due to replication errors during rapid viral reproduction and lack of RNA repair systems in host cells, nor does it exclude recombination with endogenous flaviviruses and possibility of selection of pathogenic variants. Only recombinant attenuated flaviviruses obtained by co-transfection of cell cultures with several plasmid DnA and cloned genome fragments can ensure relative safety. Mucosal immunization of mice with recombinant Gram-negative bacteria presenting on the surface and secreting nonstructural glycoprotein NS1 VCE resulted in the induction of antibodies with high titers, which did not provide protection against infection even by homologous strains of the virus. Since the variability of the viral proteins of RNA-containing flaviviruses makes it difficult to create new generation vaccines, immunogenic peptides were selected according to the criteria of their conservativity and surface localization to be presented to the immune system. One of the most conserved fragments of flavivirus proteins located on the virion surface is the "fusion peptide. Initially, a linear synthetic peptide corresponding to the conserved 98 to 113 amino acid residues (a. o.) of the E VCE protein was conjugated to snail hemocyanin KLH, and immunization of rats resulted in viral neutralizing antibodies with a high neutralization index of 3.0 (Volkova et al., 1998). In 2008, the tick-borne flavivirus fusion peptide was incorporated into multiple antigenic peptides (MAPs) modeling conformational antigenic determinants. In addition to the B-cell epitope, a fusion peptide, T-cell epitopes were incorporated into MAPs to enable a balanced immune response. Without conjugation to high-molecular-weight antigens, MAP induced antibodies with high titers capable of inhibiting hemagglutination and neutralizing VCE and other flaviviruses. The safety, low cost, chemical stability, ability to select conserved protein fragments with surface localization, high epitope density, antigenicity, and immunogenicity of MAP allow the development of approaches to prevention, medical diagnosis, and monitoring of natural populations of not only various tick-borne RNA-containing flaviviruses but also bacteria and protozoa.

4

1. Vaccination against tick-borne encephalitis

1.1. Analysis of risk, prevalence and incidence of tick-borne encephalitis

Among RNA-containing tick-borne flaviviruses, the tick-borne encephalitis virus (BTV) dominates in natural foci throughout Eurasia. Entering the human body through tick bites, VCE causes severe diseases, often with neurological, disabling or fatal consequences. Over the past 75 years, research to develop and improve methods of prevention and treatment of tick-borne encephalitis has been ongoing.

The range of tick-borne encephalitis virus (BTV) includes the taiga and mixed forest areas of Eurasia from the Pacific to the Atlantic Oceans with registration in France, northern Italy and Scandinavian countries (particularly Norway) in the west and in Northern China and Northern Japan in the east. Highly endemic areas are Austria, Slovenia, the Czech Republic, the Baltic States and Russia (for references see Mansfield et al. , 2009; Leonova, 2009). In Russia, natural outbreaks of tick-borne encephalitis have been registered from Arkhangelsk to Udmurtia and Tatarstan in the European part of Russia, in the Urals, Western and Eastern Siberia, and in the Far East (Vorobyova, 2006). In natural foci, VEE circulates as part of a parasitic system that includes the virus, its arthropod hosts (tick vectors), and vertebrate hosts (tick feeders). Formation and development of natural foci of tick-borne encephalitis depends on a complex of ecological factors, which include temperature and relative air humidity, soil moisture, features of biotope vegetation, as well as density and population dynamics of tick populations and their feeders, virulence of ticks, susceptibility to VCE and immune layer in vertebrate reservoir hosts, etc. (Lvov et al., 1989;

Korotkov et al., 2007; Hofmann, 1973; Plassmann,1980; and references in Tick-Borne Encephalitis (TBE) and its Immunoprophylaxis, 1996). It is widespread mostly within the ranges of its main vectors - ixodes ticks: 1) taiga tick - *Ixodes persulcatus*

Schulze and 2) forest tick - *Ixodes ricinus* L, what is determined by ecological conditions necessary for reproduction of virus in arthropod organisms with following biological transmission (Lvov et al., 1989).

After the discovery of TSE and improvements in diagnostic methods, data on the incidence of tick-borne encephalitis increased until it became clear that the incidence of human tick-borne encephalitis everywhere is cyclic with significant periodic rises once every 10-12 years and small peaks every 3-4 years (for references see Morozova and Bakhvalova, 2010). Maximum morbidity of the population in tick-borne encephalitis-endemic territories is observed 1-2 years, followed by a period of decline in morbidity for 1-5 years, followed by stabilization at the minimum level lasting 6-7 years and a new rise to the maximum level (Fig. 1). Cyclical changes are characteristic not only for the general level of morbidity, but also for the ratio of clinical forms. The maximum incidence was recorded in 1956, when 5,163 cases (4.5 per 100,000 population) and in 1964. (5,205 cases). Then, until 1974, there was a decrease in the incidence to 1119 cases. Since 1974 the morbidity of tick-borne encephalitis began to increase. Between 1976 and 1989, the average annual incidence of tick-borne encephalitis in Europe and Russia was 2,755 cases and, since 1990, there has been an increase by almost 400% to an average of 8,755 cases per year (Mansfield et al., 2009). In 1999 alone there were 11,356 cases of tick-borne encephalitis worldwide (www.tbe-info.com). In Russia, the maximum incidence was 10,298 in 1996 and 9,955 in 1999 (Vorobyova, 2006). These underestimates of TBE morbidity are based on the number of hospitalized patients diagnosed with encephalitis, meningoencephalitis or meningoencephalomyelitis and represent about 20-30% of the true number of people infected with TBE. The parameters traditionally used to assess the epidemic activity of natural encephalitis foci - the abundance of the main vectors, i.e., ixodid ticks, and their frequency of VEE infection - do not correlate with the levels of human morbidity in different endemic areas (for references see Morozova, Bakhvalova, 2010). Factors influencing the incidence of tick-borne encephalitis include:

1 - natural factors (solar activity, air temperature, relative humidity);

2 - population dynamics of the components of the tick-borne encephalitis parasitic system consisting of VEE, its vertebrate and invertebrate reservoir hosts;

3 - immunization against tick-borne encephalitis (Fig. 1).

Periodic variability of the incidence of tick-borne encephalitis

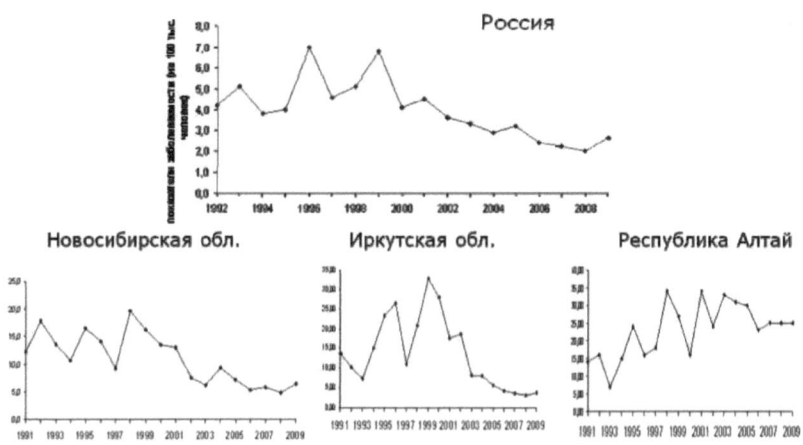

Factors affecting morbidity:
1-natural factors (solar activity, air temperature, relative humidity)
2 - population dynamics of the components of the tick-borne encephalitis parasitic system
3-immunization against tick-borne encephalitis

Fig. 1. Periodic variability of the incidence of tick-borne encephalitis

It should be noted that before mass immunization in endemic areas, virus-specific antibodies were detected in 4-8% of the population in Austria; 2-38% in the Czech Republic; 0.4-39.0% in Finland, 7-42% in Germany, and 30-100% in Russia (Tick-Borne Encephalitis (TBE) and its Immunoprophylaxis, 1996), which may indicate frequent contacts of natural foci of infection with VEE. In recent years, the real immune layer of the adult population in endemic areas of Russia has been about 40%. Thus, in 2007, in the Altai Republic, antibodies to E protein of VEE were detected in 508 (36.2%) of 1405 donors tested by ELISA (Shchuchinova, 2009).

Currently, active immunization with modern safe and 95-99% effective vaccines is the most effective way to specifically prevent tick-borne encephalitis (for references see Mansfield et al., 2009).

1.2. History of tick-borne encephalitis vaccines

Since 1930s, after the description of tick-borne encephalitis in many European countries (USSR (1932), Austria (1927), Czechoslovakia (1932), etc.) and isolation of its causative agent - VSE in 1937, the attempts to create a vaccine for active immunization of risk groups were made. The first inactivated vaccine against tick-borne encephalitis from the brains of infected mice was developed in the USSR a year after the discovery of VSE, in 1938. Of the first 29 strains of VSE isolated in the Far East in 1937 from the brains of dead patients and from the taiga tick *Ixodes persulcatus* Schulze, strain Sofyin from the brain of a patient who died in 1937 was chosen for vaccines. (for references, see Timofeev and Karganova, 2003). After 2-3 intraperitoneal injections, this vaccine protected mice against 100-10,000 LD50 VSE (for references, see Timofeev and Karganova, 2003). This effective but highly reactive vaccine was used until 1958.

Inadequate purification of the first vaccine resulted in decreased efficacy and numerous side effects. In addition to allergic complications, cases of demyelinating encephalitis were identified. Therefore, the 5% mouse brain suspension containing

8.5 lg LD50 VCE was replaced by a 2.5% brain suspension. No European strains of VSE were isolated in European countries until World War II. The first strains of VEE were isolated in Austria only in 1953, in Czechoslovakia in 1948, and in Germany only in 1974. Therefore, there were no simultaneous attempts to create European vaccines against tick-borne encephalitis. In 1958, Levkovich and Zasuchina developed a vaccine based on formaldehyde-inactivated VCE from primary culture of chicken embryo fibroblasts, and D.K. Lvov and colleagues tested a new vaccine based on the former Far East strain Sofyin. A new technology for concentrating and purifying the inactivated tick-borne encephalitis vaccine was proposed by Elbert in the 1970s and is still used today (for references see Timofeev and Karganova, 2003). In Austria, the first tick-borne encephalitis vaccine based on Nydorf strain from chicken embryo cells, partially purified by chromatography on hydroxyapatite and then inactivated with formalin was developed in 1973. The protective effect of such vaccines exceeded 99%, but elevated body temperature, fever and headache, especially after the first injection, were recorded more often in children, which were thought to be due to insufficient purification of viral antigens. Concentration and additional purification of viral antigens were achieved by centrifugation of formalin-inactivated VCE in a sucrose density gradient or by chromatography on macroporous glass. Increased concentrations of virus-specific antigens contributed to the induction of cellular immunity in vaccinated individuals, as confirmed by the blast-transformation reaction (for references, see Timofeev and Karganova, 2003). In Germany, Bock et al. first reported in 1990 on the design of a new formalin inactivated vaccine (Block et al., 1990). The high rate of adverse reactions, especially in children, led to the need to reduce the amounts of virus-specific antigens. Despite a positive correlation between amounts of VCE antigen ranging from 0.03-3.0 µg per dose and titers of induced virus-specific antibodies (Bock et al., 1990), lower amounts of VCE antigen in Encepur vaccine maintained levels of immune response with minimal incidence of complications (for references, see Timofeev and Karganova, 2003).

An alternative approach was to develop a live attenuated vaccine against tick-borne encephalitis (Mayer et al., 1967; Mayer, 1973; Smorodinthev et al., 1969). The success of the live yellow fever vaccine derived from multiple passages with high multiplicity of infection and the known greater specificity of live vaccines compared with inactivated vaccines has led to numerous attempts to select the most genetically stable Langate virus clones (strain Tp21 and its clonal isolate E5), Scottish sheep encephalomyelitis and VSE (strain Pan and Erofeev VSE isolates from ticks after passages in the spleen and liver of laboratory rats) (for references see Timofeev and Karganova, 2003). Mayer and colleagues in the Czech Republic attenuated a highly virulent strain of Chipr during persistent infection of human epithelial cell culture for 400 days followed by selection of the least virulent clone. Despite careful selection of candidate live attenuated vaccines from individual plaques, the flaviviruses recovered quasispecies heterogeneity and pathogenic properties during storage or additional passivation in chicken embryo fibroblasts, which accounted for the tragic consequences of immunization of 649479 individuals with live Dubov vaccine, of whom 35 had VCE infection resulting in meningitis and meningoencephalitis (for references, see Timofeev and Karganova, 2003).

1.3. Modern vaccines against tick-borne encephalitis

Currently, 6 types of tick-borne encephalitis vaccines similar in production technology, composition, immunization regimen, and efficacy and therefore interchangeable (Figure 2) are widely used in many European and Asian countries (Mandl et al., 1989; Vorobyova, 2006; Leonova, 2009).

Vaccines against QE permitted for use in the Russian Federation		
Name	Manufacturer	Age
EC culture purified concentrate inactivated dry vaccine	Federal State Unitary Enterprise "Perm State Research Institute of Water Problems named after M.P. Lomonosov. M.P. Chumakov Russian Academy of Medical Sciences (Russia)	From 3 years old
EnceVir	FSUE NPO Microgen M3 RF (Russia)	From 3 years old
FSME-IMMUN	Baxter AG (Austria)	From 16 years old
FSME-IMMUN Junior	Baxter AG (Austria)	1 year to 16 years
ENCEPUR adult	Novartis Vaccines and Diagnostics GmbH ft. KG (Germany)	From 12 years old
ENCEPUR for children	Novartis Vaccines and Diagnostics GmbH ft. KG (Germany)	1 to 11 years old

Fig. 2. Inactivated tick-borne encephalitis vaccines approved in Russia.

It should be noted that none of the existing vaccines have been approved by the Food and Drug Adminstrati on (FDA) for use in the United States, despite the increasing flow of tourists, U.S. military action in endemic In the production of inactivated vaccines, Russian manufacturers (the Institute of Poliomyelitis and Viral Encephalitis Institute of the Russian Academy of Medical Sciences, Moscow Region, Mikron, Russia), the Russian Institute of Poliomyelitis and Viral Encephalitis, Moscow Region, and the Russian Institute of Microbiology and Laboratory Medicine, Moscow, Russia (Arguin et al., 1999), have been instrumental in the development and production of vaccines for tick-borne encephalitis in Eurasia. In the production of inactivated vaccines, Russian manufacturers (the Institute of Poliomyelitis and Viral Encephalitis of RAMS (PIPiVE), Moscow Region, and Mikrogen (Virion NPO, Tomsk, Russia) have traditionally used strains of the vaccine. Tomsk) traditionally use VEE strains of the Far Eastern genetic type (strains Sofjin and 205, respectively), and foreign firms Baxter (Austria) and Novartis (Germany) use Western European strains Naidorf and K23, respectively (Fig. 2). In addition, 2 new vaccines against tick-borne encephalitis were developed at PIPVE of RAMS, Moscow Region, which were approved by FSUN State Research Institute of Standardization and Control of Medical Biological Preparations named after L.A. Tarasevich of Rospotrebnadzor in 2010. The new vaccines are still based on the Far Eastern strain of Sofjin VSE isolated in 1937, but differ from previous vaccines in the way they were purified and in the fact that one of the new vaccines is derived for the virus from the Vero green monkey kidney cell culture. The 0.5 ml dosage of the domestic vaccines is the same for children from 3 years old and adults. Foreign vaccines have different dosages: 0.5 ml for adults and 0.25 ml for children. All vaccines have a shelf life of 2 years. Vaccines are administered according to a similar schedule: two vaccinations with an interval of 2 to 6 months, a third one after 1 year and a revaccination after 3 to 5 years.

The characteristics of modern tick-borne encephalitis vaccines are given in Table 1. Protein antigens in tick-borne encephalitis vaccines may include BSE proteins, homologous human serum albumin, heterologous proteins of chicken embryos, and bovine serum albumin (BSA) from cell culture media and are the main reactogenicity factors. The content of VEE antigens in domestic vaccines exceeds that of for foreign analogues. Thus, the highest number of viral proteins is contained in the PIPiVE vaccine (Moscow obl.) - 4.5 µg/dose, in the vaccine Encevir (Microgen, Tomsk) - 3.5 µg/dose, in the vaccine FSME -Immun- Inject - 2.0-3,5 µg/dose for adults and half as much for children, in Encepur Adult vaccine - 1.5 µg, Encepur Children - 0.75 µg (Table 1) (Vorobyova, 2002; Leonova 2009).

Table 1: Characteristics of modern tick-borne encephalitis vaccines according to Leonova, 2009.

Vaccine name	Protein content (in µg per dose)		
	Antigen WCE	Albumin man	Squirrels chicken embryo
Encevir (Microgen, Tomsk)	3,5	250	0,5
Concentrated vaccine (PIPVE, Moscow)	4,5	250	0
FSME-IMMUN-INJECT-adult (Baxter, Austria)	2,38	500	0
FSME-IMMUN-INJECT-children (Baxter, Austria)	1,19	250	0
Encepur-adult (Novartis, Germany)	1,5	0	0
Encepur-adult (Novartis, Germany)	0,75	0	0

Due to the reactogenicity of inactivated vaccines from chicken embryonic fibroblasts, requirements for purification of vaccine preparations from foreign proteins are constantly tightening. Russian and Austrian vaccines against tick-borne encephalitis contain human albumin 250 or 500 µg in one dose, which stabilizes the viral antigen and mitigates the effect of the adjuvant, aluminum hydroxide, on the immune system (Marth and Kleinhappl, 2002; Leonova, 2009), with amounts of other ballast proteins of no more than 65 µg per dose for Encevir vaccine (Microgen) and no more than 30 for PIPiVE vaccine (Moscow). and the absence of chicken embryo proteins in most vaccines with the exception of Encevir (0.5 µg). The German tick-borne encephalitis vaccine contains no protein stabilizers (polygelin and albumin), which reduces unwanted allergic reactions and the risk of transmission of dangerous infections with human albumin from donor blood (for references see Leonova, 2009). Viral antigens are stabilized with 40-60 mg/ml sucrose. The criterion for purification of vaccines from ballast proteins can be the BSA content from culture media for VCE growth, which is regulated and monitored. For PIPiVE vaccine (Moscow), the BSA content should not exceed 0.5 µg in a 1 ml dose, which is 500 times higher than the requirements for purification of the German vaccine "Encepur" ("Baxter", Germany) (required BSA content is not more than 0.1 µg/ml, and the real content is less than 1 ng/ml).

In addition to proteins, tick-borne encephalitis vaccines contain aluminum hydroxide as an adjuvant (aluminum content 0.6-0.8 mg/ml for Encepur (Baxter, Germany) and 0.27-0.53 mg/ml in PIPiVE vaccine (Moscow). Introduction of human growth hormone into inactivated tick-borne encephalitis vaccines ensured complete protection of laboratory animals against VEE infection after a single injection, apparently through attachment of VEE antigen in complex with human growth hormone to insoluble aluminum hydroxide matrix and subsequent clonal expansion of antigen-specific T lymphocytes that migrated to such supramolecular complexes at injection sites (Stephenson et al, 1991). However, additional adjuvants (cytokines, immunomodulators, and other biologically active substances) in inactivated vaccines have not been widely used so far because of the unpredictable long-term consequences of interference with the immune response.

Comparative studies of the efficacy and safety of tick-borne encephalitis vaccines registered in the Russian Federation (Fig. 2) showed that the frequencies of seroconversions for the vaccines Encevir (Microgen, Tomsk) (74.6-98.6%), PIPiVE (58.8-99.2%), FSME-IMMUN (Austria) (21.8-96.6%) and Encepur (Germany) (14.0-

95.0%) (the first figure corresponds to the proportion of seropositive to VSE sera after the first vaccination, and the second one after the third vaccination) and average antibody titers against VEE did not differ significantly, but as a result of double immunization with FSME-IMMUN vaccine (Austria) antibody titers over 1:1600 detected more frequently (Prokhorova et al., 2006), which does not directly correlate with VEE antigen concentrations (Table 1). Reactogenicity and changes in blood biochemical parameters are related to the method of vaccine administration. Viral carriage without clinical manifestations is not a contraindication for vaccination. At present, Encevir vaccine (Microgen, Tomsk) is the optimal preparation for mass immunization in terms of price-quality ratio, which is confirmed by the data on the ratio of vaccines used against tick-borne encephalitis in endemic areas of Russia, among which domestic vaccines certainly prevail, of which Encevir is at least 60%.

Austria had the highest incidence of tick-borne encephalitis in Europe (up to 700 hospitalized cases annually) (Fig. 3). After the introduction of mass vaccination against tick-borne encephalitis in 1981, the incidence rate dropped dramatically. In Austria, 88% of the population was vaccinated, of which only 58% had no violation of the recommended immunization regimen, with morbidity reduced to sporadic cases only among unvaccinated persons (Fig. 3). Vaccine efficacy is more than 95%, i.e., vaccination is able to prevent at least 95 out of 100 cases of tick-borne encephalitis. However, with the exception of Austria, immunization success in other endemic areas is not so clear, since vaccines are relatively expensive and require repeated injections to maintain protective immunity (Mansfield et al., 2009). In comparison, neighboring Western European countries with similar climatic conditions have seen increases in tick-borne encephalitis incidence with vaccination coverage rates of 11% in the Czech Republic (Figure 3), 13% in Germany and 6% in Lithuania (for references see Leonova, 2009).

NUMBER OF QE CASES IN AUSTRIA AND THE CZECH REPUBLIC AND VACCINATION RATES IN AUSTRIA

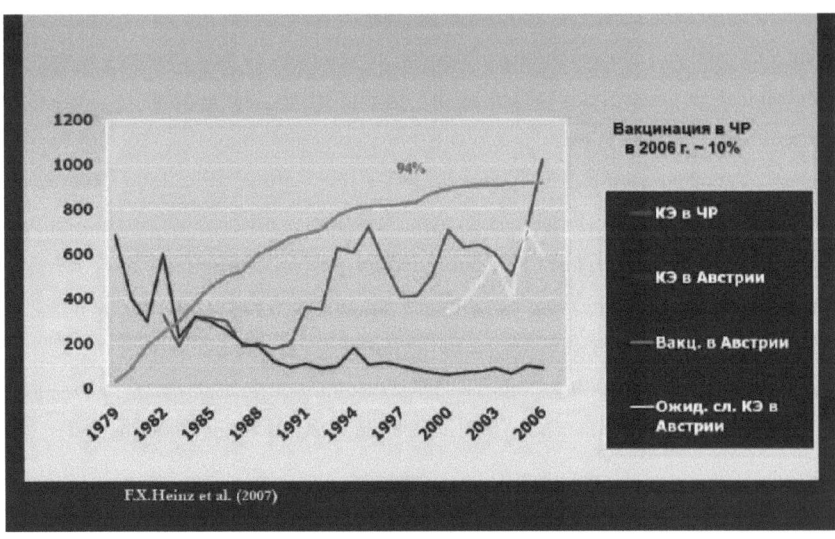

Figure 3. Vaccination and morbidity rates for tick-borne encephalitis in Austria and the Czech Republic (Heinz *et al.,* 2007).

In the Russian Federation, between 2.5 and 3 million people are immunized and revaccinated annually. At the same time until now the coverage of the population with immunization against tick-borne encephalitis is on average 5-7% (Fig. 4), in spite of 6 types of vaccines approved for use in the Russian Federation (Fig. 2). Therefore, the low immunization coverage does not affect the periodically changing incidence of tick-borne encephalitis among the population of endemic regions of Russia (Fig. 5).

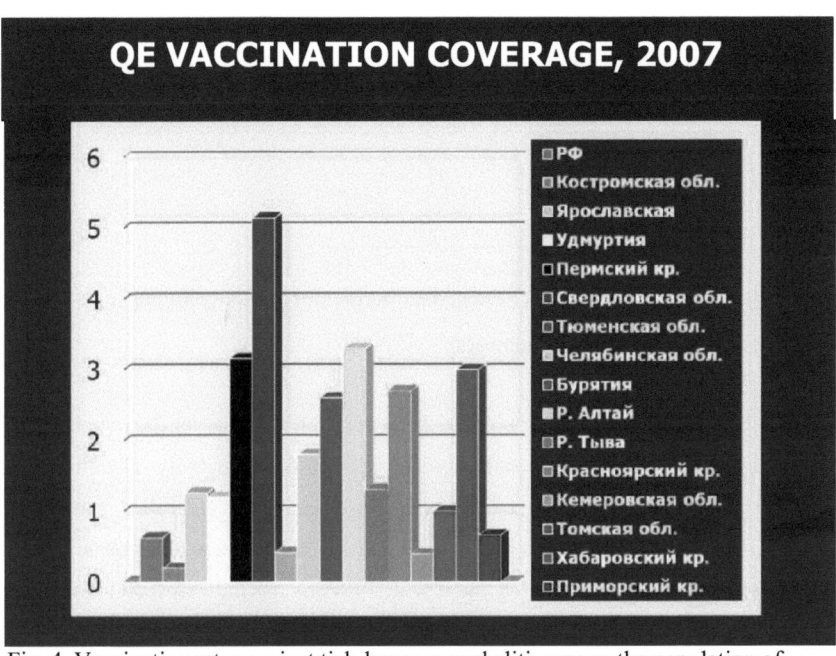

Fig. 4. Vaccination rates against tick-borne encephalitis among the population of endemic regions of Russia.

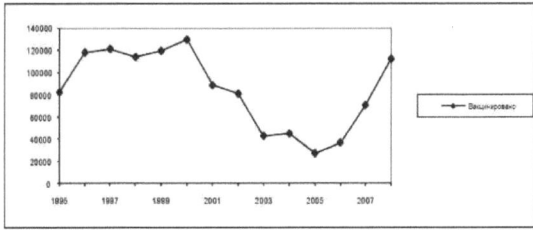

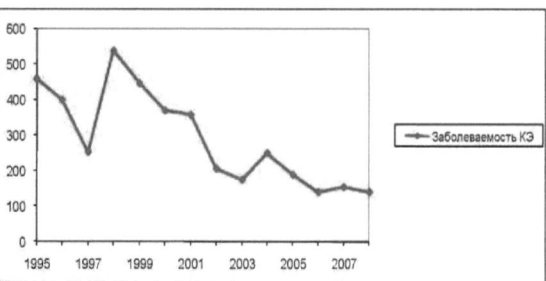

Fig. 5. Dynamics of vaccination rates and morbidity of tick-borne encephalitis in the Novosibirsk Region (absolute numbers).

The use of primary cultures of chicken embryo fibroblasts for the reproduction of vaccine strains of VEE ensures the absence of carcinogenic activity. Therefore, the nucleic acid content of modern inactivated vaccines is not controlled. However, cytokine activities (interleukins 10, 2, 4, 6, 10, 12, tumor necrosis factor a and y-interferon) after immunization of mice with PIPiVE vaccine (Moscow) testify to activation of macrophages, T- and B-lymphocytes (Ignatyev et al, 2003), which is not typical for purified proteins, which are exogenous antigens and therefore induce immune response through Th-2 pathway with secretion of inteleukins 4 and 5, but not y-interferon (Sartakova, Konenkov, 1997). Quantification of VCE RNA in Encevir vaccine (Microgen, Tomsk) by the Schmidt-Tannhauser method (for references, see Morozova et al, 2006) and fractionation in 2M LiCl revealed more resistant to the action of RNA-ases double-stranded RNAs, characteristic of replicative forms and partially for replicative intermediates of RNA-containing flaviviruses, and trace amounts of single-stranded RNAs. Determination of nucleotide sequences of reverse transcription products followed by PCR showed 900 np long fragments of the VCE genome of vaccine strain 205 (for references, see Morozova et al., 2006). Quantification by real-time PCR with a fluorescent probe showed threshold cycles of at least 40 (Fig. 6) corresponding to single genome-equivalents of VCE in the reaction mixture, which, taking into account the efficiency of RNA isolation and reversion as well as aliquots for analysis at each stage, allowed us to estimate the content of 10-100 copies of viral RNA in 1 ml of Encevir vaccine.

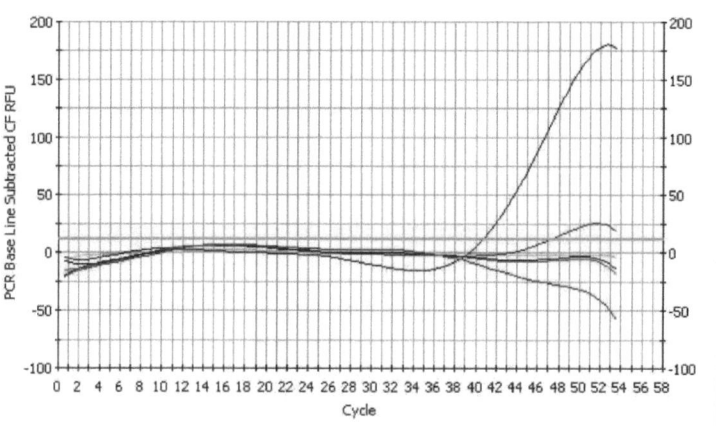

Figure 6. Nucleic acid analysis in Encevir vaccine (Microgen) by reverse transcription followed by real-time PCR with primers and fluorescent probe corresponding to the NS1 gene of the Far Eastern type of VEE.

Double-stranded RNAs are known to enhance the synthesis of different types of interferons and increase the functional activity of macrophages and neutrophils. Double-stranded RNAs in Encevir vaccine with a length of more than 30 bp can induce interferon synthesis, while 20-25 bp can induce RNA interference (for references, see Morozova et al., 2006). It should be noted that the presence of cDNA in tick-borne encephalitis vaccines in the absence of DNA stage in the replication of RNA-containing flaviviruses may be a consequence of retroviral revertase activity during reproduction of VCE in chicken embryo fibroblasts, which should be carefully controlled due to the emerging risk of genetic rearrangements resulting from the possible integration of DNA copies of VCE genome fragments into cell chromosomes. Thus, the presence of viral nucleic acids in inactivated vaccine preparations and cellular nucleic acids can probably induce balanced cellular and humoral immunity for effective elimination of VCE-infected cells and extracellular virions and requires regulated monitoring.

Traditional technologies for producing inactivated vaccines based on developing chicken embryos currently cannot meet public health needs. Since 1995, the World Health Organization (WHO) has recommended that vaccines should not be developed using chicken embryos as a substrate, but rather transplanted cell cultures certified in accordance with international requirements for cell substrates (WHO Cell Culture, 1995; Sheets and Petricciani, 2004). Such cell cultures have several advantages: 1) the ability to be cultured in systems with a developed surface (in rollers and bioreactors), in serum-free or serum-reduced media; 2) the stability of properties over long periods of time to work with vaccine strains; and 3) the ability to produce viral biomass of vaccine strains with unchanged antigenic properties (WHO Cell Culture, 1995; Sheets and Petricciani, 2004). However, grafted cell cultures can accumulate foreign agents from nutrient media, sera, trypsin, etc. during serial passaging. The use of any cell culture carries the risk of contamination with viruses or mycoplasmas. The use of grafted cell lines for vaccine production requires a reduction of cellular DNA concentrations to the WHO-limited level of no more than 100 pg per dose, which reduces the risk of transforming activity.

To compare the reproduction of vaccine-derived and isolated VEE strains in 2009 and 2010 in various permissive cell cultures, cells of embryonic SPEV and Vero (B) and Vero E6 green monkey kidney cells were infected with 6 different VEE strains isolated from tick-borne encephalitis patients (Sophin and Aina strains) or from ticks (strains 205, 2530, 2689 and 2703). The choice of strains was determined by the predominance of the Siberian and Far East types of VEE in most natural foci of Russia and neighboring countries. The strains of the Far East genetic type included the strain Sofyin VSE isolated from the brain of a dead patient in the Far East in 1937; and strain 205 isolated from the tick *I. persulcatus* in Khabarovsk Territory in 1973. Strains of Siberian genetic type included the strain Ain, isolated from a patient in Irkutsk Region in 1963. , and strains 2530, 2689, and 2703 isolated from *I. persulcatus* ticks in Novosibirsk Region in 2009-10. Three strains: Sofjin, Aina, and 205 have been well studied after numerous passages in SPEV cell culture and in the brain of laboratory mice, and are probably phylogenetic precursors of the modern biodiversity of viral isolates. Three freshly isolated strains have been studied at the level of initial infection in sucker mice and reflect the current stage of VCE evolution. All 6 strains have never been previously adapted to Vero cells. After infection of transplanted cell cultures, viable VCE titers reached 2.8 lg CPD50 for Vero (B) cells, 5.5 lg CPD50 for Vero E6 and up to 9 lg CPD50 for SPEV cells. Quantitative assessments of E VCE antigen by enzyme immunoassay and genome equivalents by reverse transcription followed by real-time PCR allowed us to estimate up to 10^8 virions in 1 ml of culture liquid, which corresponded to microscopic CPD observations for SPEV cells and significantly exceeded those for Vero E6 cells and especially for Vero (B) cells. Based on the data of VCE strain titration, ELISA and real-time RT-PCR, the domestic vaccine line Vero (B), characterized according to the WHO requirements, and Vero E6 cells can be used for the development of vaccines against tick-borne encephalitis.

The protective effect of the domestic inactivated vaccines was studied in BALB/c mice (females, weight 14-16 g) against the highly virulent strain VKE 396 (GenBank access number DQ394880) isolated from *I. persulcatus* tick in 1981. The highly virulent strain 2530 (GU060547) also isolated from a taiga tick in Novosibirsk in 1981, but with low morbidity of TBE (8.87 cases per 100,000 persons) in 2009. Mice were immunized with domestic vaccines subcutaneously 3 times in 0.5 ml of diluted 1:10, 1:32, 1:100 and 1:320 vaccines with 7-day intervals between injections. Seven days after the last vaccine injection, mice were injected intraperitoneally with VCE 100 and 1000 LD50/0.25 mL. At 90% lethality in the control groups, the lethality of the vaccinated mice was 37.5% and 31.2% in the groups infected with 1000 and 100 LD50, respectively. The significance of differences according to Student's test was 0.01. In the group of vaccinated mice infected with 1000 LD50 of VKE strain 396, the average life span was 34 days, while in the control group it was 13 days (I=2.6). In the experimental and control groups with a dose of 100 LD50 VKE, the mean life expectancy was 45 and 13 days, respectively (I=3.4). The resistance index, defined as the ratio of virus titers in groups of vaccinated and intact animals of equal weight, age and lineage, was 4.8 lg LD50. The titers of virus-neutralizing antibodies ranged from 1.225 to 1.45 lg (data provided by Anufrieva E.A. (Institute of Systematics and Ecology of Animals SB RAS, Novosibirsk). No tick-borne encephalitis symptoms were detected among the mice immunized with Encevir vaccine produced by Tomsk Microgen Ltd. in dilutions from 1:10 to 1:32 and then infected with strain 2530 of Siberian genetic type VSE. Signs of tick-borne encephalitis were noted in the group of mice immunized with Encevir vaccine at a dilution of 1:100. Thus, despite the induction of a predominantly humoral immune response after administration of exogenous antigens of inactivated vaccines (Sartakova and Konenkov, 1997), the presence of large amounts of all denatured viral proteins in inactivated tick-borne encephalitis vaccines resulted in protection against VEE of the Far Eastern and Siberian genetic types that dominate in Russia and the near abroad, including the 2009 VEE strain of isolation.

However, current vaccines are not ideal. Side effects of vaccines include fever above ^{380C} and fever in over 1% of children and neurological complications in adults. Reducing the dose of VEE antigens by a factor of 2-4 in the Western European childhood vaccines FSME-IMMUN-INJECT-children (Baxter, Austria) and Encepur (Novartis, Germany) (Table 1) reduces the risk of complications, most of which are due to the ability of inactivated viral particles to stimulate the cytokine response, especially inducing expression of tumor necrosis factor TNF-a and interleukin IL-10 genes (Marth and Kleinhappl, 2002). Massive complications in children after immunization with the Encevir vaccine produced by NPO Microgen in the summer of 2010 led to the ban of this childhood vaccine in the Russian Federation.

The limited protective effect of inactivated vaccines and the relatively short immunological memory are caused mainly by the humoral immune response. Glycoprotein E of flaviviruses is a relatively weak inducer of cytotoxic T cells because it causes the development of an immune response through the Tb2 pathway (Timofeev et al., 1998). Levels of virus-neutralizing antibodies with predominance of IgG2a immunoglobulins were higher after administration of live or recombinant virus compared to immunization with recombinant E protein, after which IgG1 immunoglobulins prevail (Timofeev et al., 1998).

In addition, flaviviruses are known to have the effect of enhancing infection through pre-existing antibodies (antibody-dependent enchancement), whereby a strong immune response causes pathological consequences for the organism in secondary infection, leading to a decrease in the average lifetime and death of immunized animals after infection (Peiris and Porterfield, 1979; Phillpotts et al. , 1985). Immune complexes of virions with specific antibodies penetrate into monocytes through the Fc-receptor, leading to an increase in the total number of infected cells and, consequently, a more productive infection against the background of immunosuppression. At the same time, cytokine concentrations and lymphocyte counts increase, leading to a cascade increase in the level of infectivity of the organism. The effect of immune enhancement of flavivirus infectivity (antibody-dependent enhancement) is epitope specific and is not induced by any MCA directed to glycoprotein E (Phillpotts et al. , 1985). It is possible that immune enhancement of infectivity is caused both by penetration of virion complexes with antibodies to glycoprotein E into monocytes and macrophages as a result of binding to the Fc-receptor (Thomas, 1993) and by activation of RNA synthesis as a result of binding of the RNA-matrix shielding structural protein of virions E (Morozova et al. , 1990).

Despite 95-99% effective protection against infection with homologous strains of VEE (for references see, e.g., Tick-Borne Encephalitis (TBE) and its Immunoprophylaxis. Tick-Borne Encephalitis (TBE) and its Immunoprophylaxis, 1996; Timofeev and Karganova, 2003; Vorobyeva, 2002; Leonova 2009; Mansfield et al., 2009), the available vaccines do not provide complete protection against infection with heterologous virus strains belonging to evolutionarily distant genetic types of VEE. The paradox is that high immunization rates in the Sverdlovsk Region (in 2010, 78% of the population) and in the Altai Republic (40% of the population) (Fig. 4) coincide with high morbidity rates, exceeding the Russian average by 2-6 and 10 times, respectively. Immunization of the population against tick-borne encephalitis in the Altai Republic is carried out mainly with Encevir vaccine produced by NPO Microgen. In recent years the immunization rate has been 40.0±0.2% of the population. At the same time, the real immune layer of the adult population was 36.1±2.5% (Shchuchinova, 2009).

In addition, vaccination does not always prevent the disease. In Primorsky Krai,

15.1% of persons vaccinated against tick-borne encephalitis in the 1990s and 8.2% of persons vaccinated against tick-borne encephalitis in the 2000s recorded the disease with mortality rates of 5.3 and 0%, respectively (Leonova, 2009). In the Altai Republic, according to long-term data, 22.7±3.3% of tick-borne encephalitis patients were vaccinated (of which only 5.0±1.8% had a violation of the immunization scheme). However, for the immunized persons the incidence is 2 times lower and milder febrile forms of tick-borne encephalitis are characteristic (Shchuchinova, 2009).

Possible reasons for incomplete protection of immunized humans against VEE infection are genetic heterogeneity of the VEE quasispecies, mismatch between genetic types of vaccine strains and virus isolates currently dominating in natural foci of most endemic regions of Russia and the near abroad, and evolutionary changes in VEE over the past 40-70 years since vaccine strains were isolated. Characterization of VEE strains and natural isolates by serological and molecular genetic methods, including molecular hybridization of viral genomic RNA with oligonucleotide probes, determination of nucleotide sequences of the viral genome and its fragments followed by phylogenetic analysis and real-time PCR with fluorescent probes showed 3 types of VEE - Far Eastern, Siberian, and Western European (Pogodina et al., 1981; 1981a; Ecker et al., 1999; Bakhvalova et al., 2000; Zlobin et al. 1996; 2001). Exogenous presentation of viral antigens in inactivated vaccines leads to induction of a preferential humoral immune response through the type 2 T-helper pathway. The long scheme of three-times immunization and the necessity of revaccination every three years determine the search for new ways to prevent not only tick-borne encephalitis with the induction of predominantly cellular immunity by Th1 pathway, but also other flavivirus infections ecologically associated with ticks.

1.4. Adjuvants

In the 1920s, in the treatment of infectious diseases, it was discovered that adding certain substances to antigen solutions resulted in increased antibody formation. Such substances were called adjuvants. The action of adjuvants is due to their ability to retain and accumulate antigen for long-term presentation to the immune system (depot effect) or their ability to regulate the cytokine response. Aluminum salts act as a depot, inducing the formation of small granulomas in which they are retained together with the adsorbed antigen. Liposomes and immunostimulatory complexes (ISCOMs) also depot antigen, while adjuvants of bacterial origin, mainly cell walls of killed bacteria, stimulate the formation of corresponding cytokines. Cytokines are more effective when bound to the antigen. The use of cytokines is useful in vaccinating immunocompromised individuals for whom the conventional vaccines are not effective enough. It is possible that the use of cytokines can regulate the development of an immune response through the Th1 or Th2 pathway.

Currently, there is a large number of immunomodulators of microbial, plant, synthetic and mineral origin, differing in origin and mechanism of adjuvant action. It is known that the action of many adjuvants is mediated through the induction of synthesis of various cytokines capable of influencing the formation of specific and nonspecific immune response. Thus, adjuvants of microbial origin (muramyldipeptide, lipid A) induce the production of interleukin-1 (IL-1), immunomodulator of synthetic origin (Avridin) - synthesis of IL-1 and interferon-gamma (IFNy). All this points to the possibility of natural replacement of a number of adjuvants by cytokine preparations. There are reports on the use of cytokines such as IL-1, IL-2, IFNy, granulocyte-macrophage colony-stimulating factor (GM-CSF), tumor necrosis factor a (TNFa) in vaccinations against hepatitis B, rabies, malaria, herpes. Other vaccines use both inorganic salts (particularly aluminum phosphate and calcium phosphate) and bacterial products (whole-cell killed pertussis vaccine) as adjuvants. To enhance the cellular immune response, cytokines IL-1, IL-2, IL-12, and interferon gamma, as well as liposomes, copolymers for penetration of antigenic complexes into immune system cells to present antigens from cells, sustained-release drugs, and immunostimulatory complexes, are attempted to be added to vaccines, but they are all in the experimental stage of development and are not yet approved for vaccination of the population.

At present, aluminum hydroxide is used as an adjuvant in tick-borne encephalitis vaccines. There have also been attempts to stimulate the specific immune response in tick-borne encephalitis using an inducer of interferon synthesis RFf2, which was accompanied by a significant increase in the overall resistance of animals during their subsequent infection (Avdeeva et al., 2009). In experiments on mice the stimulating effect of a number of cytokines on the immunogenic activity of the tick-borne encephalitis vaccine was established. The most pronounced effect was exerted by recombinant IL-ip, human TNFa, immunophan and hybrid protein neotime (Ta-TNF-Ta), which increased the immunogenicity of the vaccine by 1.3-1.5 times (Avdeeva et al. , 2009). An increase in the immunogenicity of the vaccine was also noted when using a complex of recombinant human cytokines IL-1B, IL-2 and TNFa. The cytokine preparations under study increased the protective effect of tick-borne encephalitis vaccines as assessed by the level of resistance of BALB/c mice to infection with the VEE Absettars strain compared to the animals immunized with a single vaccine (Avdeeva et al. , 2009).

However, the replacement of cell lines and vaccine strains of VEE in accordance with WHO requirements and the current epidemiological situation in most endemic areas of Eurasia, as well as the introduction of adjuvants do not eliminate the fundamental limitations of inactivated vaccines. Therefore, further research is required on new approaches to creating vaccines with broad specificity to various flaviviruses from natural foci of infection.

2. New Approaches to Vaccines Against Tick-borne Encephalitis

New directions for the prevention of flavivirus infections based on the use of recombinant DNA, RNA and proteins, bacteria and viruses, and synthetic peptides are currently being developed. To compare the efficacy, stability, and safety of new experimental vaccines, it is necessary to study them in a single model and compare the results with traditional immunization methods.

1.1. Genetic immunization

Gene immunization is based on the introduction of plasmid DNA with infectious agent genes into the body, gene expression and presentation of antigens by transfected cells to induce an immune response (Cohen, 1993). Candidate DNA vaccines use a cellular protein-synthesizing machinery to synthesize antigens (Brower, 1998). The undoubted advantages of gene immunization are the simplicity and cheapness of obtaining DNA vaccines. The use of plasmid vectors to clone various viral genes under the control of strong promoters recognized by eukaryotic RNA polymerases greatly simplifies the method of production and reduces the time required to develop potential vaccines. In addition to promoters, such vector systems must contain ori-replications for bacterial cells and sometimes ori-replications for eukaryotic DNA-dependent DNA polymerases, antibiotic resistance gene(s) for selection on selective media, and multiple cloning sites with unique recognition sites for restriction endonucleases. No need to work with pathogenic viruses or bacteria and no expensive antigen purification procedure can significantly reduce the cost of recombinant DnA vaccines.

Since RNA-containing viruses are characterized by high genome variability (Steinhauer and Holland, 1987; Tsilinski, 1988), the viral genes in recombinant plasmids must be conserved to provide protection against a variety of natural isolates (Cohen, 1993). The most conserved flavivirus genes are E (42% homology among various species of the genus *Flavivirus)*, NS1 (42%), NS3 (44%), and NS5 (55%) (Pletnev et al., 1990). Other nonstructural proteins and nucleocapsid C protein are more variable. However, all nonstructural VCE proteins except NS1 are found inside infected cells, and the presence of surface viral antigens in vaccines is desirable for presentation of viral antigens to the host immune system and induction of protective immunity. The glycoproteins prM and E of VCE are on the surface of virions, and the glycoprotein NS1 is on the surface of infected cells (Heinz and Mandl, 1993). The E virion envelope glycoprotein induces the formation of virus-neutralizing antibodies (Monath, 1986; Timofeev et al., 1998). NS1 glycoprotein, the only nonstructural protein among the flaviviruses, is found inside and on the surface of infected cells; in addition, it is secreted as homo- and hetero-oligomeric complexes. Antibodies directed to the NS1 protein protect animals against lethal doses of flaviviruses through complement-dependent lysis of infected cells (Schlesinger et al., 1985). The nonstructural protein NS3 of VCE is required late in the infection for genomic RNA synthesis, hence, its presence in cells transfected with recombinant DNA immediately after infection could cause disruption of the replicative complex structure. The phenomenon of resistance of cells containing viral replicases to infection with homologous viruses has been previously described for plants (Carr and Zaitlin, 1993; Palukaitis and Zaitlin, 1997). Because flavivirus infections and immunization with live attenuated vaccines result in induction of CD8 cytotoxic T lymphocytes and antibodies directed to the antigenic determinants of the viral E, NS1-NS2A, and NS3 proteins, these nonstructural proteins are recommended for inclusion in subunit vaccines (Mathew et al., 1996). Therefore, after determining the primary genome structures of VKE vaccine strains (Mandl et al., 1989; Pletnev et al., 1990; Safronov et al., 1991), their respective genes were cloned in eukaryotic expression vectors to study the protective properties of prM, E, NS1, and NS3 VKE proteins. There were four recombinant plasmid DnA - pSVK3-ENS1, pSVK3- E, pSVK3-prME, and pcDNAI-NS3 - were constructed.

Delivery of DnA to animals is possible by various methods: intramuscular, intravenous, subcutaneous and intradermal injections, intranasal and oral administration. However, ballistic transfection based on bombardment of the skin with gold particles 1-3 microns in diameter coated with DNA under high helium pressure provides an optimal balance between DNA delivery to the skin epidermal cells, presentation of the antigen by dendritic cells and macrophages and rapid excretion of transfected cells at sloughing of horny skin epithelium while maintaining the protective immune response (Tang et al., 1992; Sundaram et al., 1996). Interestingly, removal of a skin section 24 h after ballistic transfection prevents the appearance of specific antibodies and cytotoxic T lymphocytes, while removal of a muscle fragment 10 min after injection does not (Raz et al., 1994; Debabov, 1997). Cationic liposomes such as lipofectin or N-[1-(2,3-dioleoyloxy)propyl]-N, N, N-trimethylammonium methyl sulfate (DOTAP) are used to increase the efficiency of DNA delivery to target cells. For oral immunization, DNA is encapsulated in microspheres consisting of polylactide-coglycoside (Gendon, 1999).

When ingested into the tissues of a living organism, foreign DnA is capable of inducing an immune response. However, high-molecular-weight DnA molecules are weak immunogens due to their mobile conformation in solution (Schwartz, 1988). In the sera of unimmunized animals, there are autoantibodies to DnA predominantly in the B-conformation, which are directed to the sugar-phosphate backbone. These antibodies belong mainly to the IgG2 class, are unable to bind complement and are characterized by low specificity. However, DNA in the Z-conformation is capable of inducing a stronger immune response. The highest antibody titers have been detected against DNA from bacteria on the skin, such as *Micrococcus lysodeikticus* and *Staphylococcus epidermidis*. The DNA of microorganisms inhabiting mucous membranes is the least antigenic (Schwartz, 1988). It turned out that vertebrate genomes differ from the primary DNA structures of bacteria, fungi, and invertebrates by the reduced content of the CpG dinucleotide (Karlin et al., 1994). The palindromic hexamer 5'- PuPuCpGPyPy3', where Pu is the purine nucleotide residue and Py is the pyrimidine nucleotide residue, is considered to be the classic "motif" that distinguishes bacterial DNA from the vertebrate genome, but variations are possible. At least 60% of vertebrate CpG dinucleotides are methylated at the 5 position of the cytosine residue, which is thought to be necessary for X chromosome inactivation and epigenetic regulation of gene expression. Further, enzymatic deamination of 5-methylcytosine can lead to TpG/CpA transcription, which is not recognized by the repair system. The absence of a specific methylase in bacteria, fungi, and invertebrates eliminates cytosine methylation and the possibility of nucleotide substitution, which makes normal CpG dinucleotide distribution possible. Thus, differences in the size, primary structures, and degree of methylation of bacterial and vertebrate DnA determine the antigenic properties of plasmid DnA isolated from bacterial cells *of Escherichia coli* (Karlin et al., 1994).

In addition to the induction of antibody formation, DNA stimulates the proliferation of B-lymphocytes (Schwartz, 1988). Methylation of bacterial DnA eliminates its mitogenic effect. The immunomodulatory properties of DNA are due to the sequential induction of cytokines, including interleukin IL-12, interferon □ , which cause activation of natural killer cells (Schwartz, 1988). Injection of bacterial DNA or oligonucleotides leads to increased levels of tumor necrosis factor (TNFG) gene expression and sensitization of macrophages (Sparwasser et al., 1997).

Mice were intramuscularly immunized 4 times every 1 week with 100 μg of plasmid vectors pSVK3 or pcDNAI, or 100 μg of recombinant plasmids pSVK3-ENS1, pSVK3-E, pSVK3-prME or pcDNAI- NS3, containing corresponding cloned VKE genes (Sophien strain). Injection of plasmid DNA into animals can lead to the appearance of antibodies in sera both to the DNA and to the foreign proteins encoded by that DNA. Autoantibodies against DNA were detected in sera of intact animals by enzyme immunoassay with average titers of 1:100. Repeated injections of 100 μg of plasmid DNA did not result in a significant increase in DNA antibody titers. Such antibodies appeared to be weakly specific and capable of recognizing both bacterial and eukaryotic DNA. Experiments showed the presence of antibodies directed to plasmid, bacterial and eukaryotic DnA in all sera studied. Introduction of recombinant plasmid DNA into living organism tissues did not change antibody titers against DNA, since DNA molecules are known to be weak immunogens due to their unstable mobile conformation in solution, which does not depend on the nucleotide sequence (Schwartz, 1988). The immunostimulatory effect of bacterial genomic and plasmid DNA with CpG motifs (Karlin et al., 1994) was probably not caused by an increase in antibodies to the DNA. Small amounts of antibodies directed to DNA are unable to bind all molecules of injected recombinant plasmids. Consequently, nucleic acids may be present in the body immediately after administration, leading to their possible uptake by host cells.

The mechanism of DnA penetration into the cells of the immunized organism is not clear enough. Cell transfection of ring DnA occurs 50-100 times better than that of linear DnA, apparently due to the more compact packing of the former (Debabov, 1997). DNA is best absorbed by myocytes, probably due to the large surface area and the presence of numerous nuclei in the periphery of the cell, the sarcoplasmic reticulum, and the system of transverse tubules (Wolff et al., 1990). When purified DNA is injected into muscle, 0.01% to 1% of transverse striated muscle cells are transformed. Regenerating muscles capture DNA more intensively, probably due to the greater accessibility of myocytes in the absence of intercellular structures. Cell transfection in the postmitotic stage is more effective (Debabov, 1997). Intramuscularly injected DNA spreads inside the muscle, is able to diffuse into the intercellular space, pass through the outer sheath and enter the myofibers (Wolff et al., 1992).

The efficiency of nucleic acid penetration into cells has been shown to differ depending on the type of cell culture (Krieg et al., 1991; Nakai et al., 1996). A study of the rate of oligodeoxyribonucleotide penetration into eukaryotic cells showed that this process is saturable and temperature dependent (Loke et al., 1989). One to two hours after incubation of oligodeoxyribonucleotides with cell cultures at 370C, the binding level reaches a plateau (Vlassov et al., 1995). Receptor-mediated endocytosis is a probable mechanism of nucleic acid entry into cells, since known endocytosis inhibitors reduce the efficiency of such transport. Methods of affinity labeling of proteins with reactive oligodeoxyribonucleotide derivatives showed the existence of two oligonucleotide-binding proteins with molecular weights of about 79 and 90 kDa on the surface of mouse fibroblasts (Yakubov et al., 1989; Loke et al., 1989) in the number of about [105] per cell (Vlassov et al., 1995). Since both RNA and single-stranded and double-stranded DNA competitively inhibited the binding of these cellular proteins to oligonucleotides, the receptors are probably common to all nucleic acids (Yakubov et al., 1989; Loke et al., 1989; Krieg et al., 1991). In addition, a protein with a molecular weight of about 30 kDa, which is involved in plasmid DNA penetration into cells, was found on the cell surface (Loke et al., 1989). In addition to specific receptors for nucleic acids, reactive oligonucleotide analogues were found to be able to interact with many proteins on the cell surface, in particular with CD4 cell receptors (Vlassov et al., 1995).

The persistence of plasmid DnA in dividing cells depends on its resistance to DnAases and the ability of plasmids to extrachromosomal replication encoded by the initiation ori replication site (Yates et al., 1985). The resistance of superspiralized plasmids to the action of nucleases depends on the type of transfected eukaryotic cells. For example, 24 h after intramuscular injection the amount of plasmid DNA becomes indeterminate in the immunized organism, while during intradermal injection DNA is present for up to 28 days (Winegar et al., 1996). When DNA is delivered intravenously using cationic liposomes, plasmids are detected for 9 weeks (Zhu et al., 1993), and when injected directly into the spleen, for 12 weeks only in spleen cells and absent in other organs (Xiong et al., 1997). However, as early as 48 hours after transfection of eukaryotic cells, mutations appeared in plasmid DNA (MacGregor et al., 1987), mostly in transplanted cell lines with decreased ability to repair (Finn et al., 1989). In addition to degradation of exogenous DnA in eukaryotic cells under the action of nucleases and appearance of mutations in them, disappearance of non-replicating plasmids due to sequential decrease of their relative amounts in the process of eukaryotic cell division is possible.

Stability of plasmids in transfected eukaryotic cells was studied *in vitro* and *in vivo*. The main targets for the introduction of plasmid DNA during gene immunization are muscle, skin, liver, kidney, spleen, and blood. Therefore, homogenates of these organs and tissues, as well as cell culture lysates at equal concentrations of total proteins determined spectrophotometrically at 280 nm were used to evaluate plasmid stability. The results of electrophoresis in 1% agarose gel followed by ethidium bromide staining of plasmid DNA after incubation with eukaryotic cell lysates showed that plasmid DNA in muscle tissue and serum was the least stable (Fig. 7).

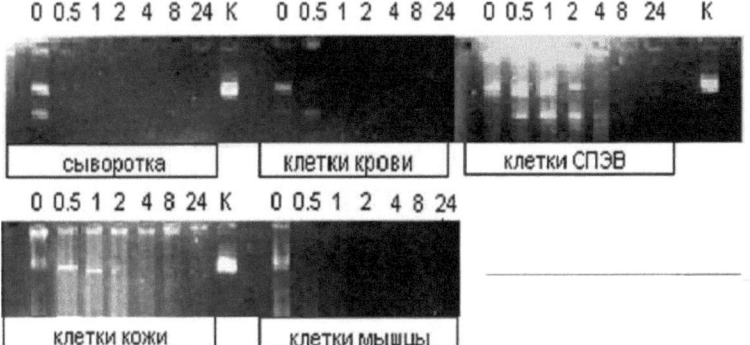

0 0.5 1 2 4 8 24 K   0 0.5 1 2 4 8 24   0 0.5 1 2 4 8 24   K

сыворотка   клетки крови   клетки СПЭВ

0 0.5 1 2 4 8 24 K   0 0.5 1 2 4 8 24

клетки кожи   клетки мышцы

Figure 7. Comparative analysis of stability of recombinant plasmid DNA pSVK3-ENS1 in serum and homogenates of blood, skin, and muscle cells and in a lysate of pig embryonic kidney cells of SPEV *in vitro*. Track numbers correspond to the incubation time of DNA with cell homogenates or lysates and serum (in hours), track K is the original plasmid.

After a 30-minute incubation of plasmids with muscle homogenates and sera, the amount of DnA becomes below the detection level of the 0.01 μg method. This is probably due to the high content of nucleases in muscle tissue and blood sera. The source of nucleases in blood serum can be products of platelet destruction, the concentration of DNAases in which is 10 times higher than in other blood cells (Shapot, 1968). Low stability of superspiralized plasmid DnA was also found in lysates of liver, kidney, and spleen cells (data not presented). DNA is more stable in lysates of blood cells, skin cells, and cell cultures, where it persists for 1-2 hours (Fig. 7). Leukocytes are known to contain DNA-ase inhibitor, which affects the stability of exogenous plasmids (Shapot, 1968). The low stability of plasmid DNA in eukaryotic cell lysates could be the result of lysosome disruption with the release of the nucleases contained in them, which does not occur in living cells. Therefore, the next step was to study plasmid resistance *in vivo*. BALB/c mice were immunized intramuscularly with 100 µg of plasmid DNA and after 10 and 24 h the plasmids isolated from the injection site were analyzed using three independent methods: electrophoresis in agarose gel, transformation of competent bacterial cells and polymerase chain reaction (PCR). The sensitivity limit for plasmid DNA detection in the agarose gel after staining with ethidium bromide under UV irradiation is 10 ng, or approximately 10^9 DNA molecules about 7,000 np long. The plasmid was detected 10 h after injection, but after 24 h its amount was below the sensitivity level of this method. The transformation of *Escherichia coli* cells with the level of 10^3 clones per 1 µg of plasmid using plasmid DNA isolated from the muscle 10 h after immunization revealed single clones that were absent when cells were transformed with plasmid DNA isolated 24 h after intramuscular injection. The data obtained indicated the presence of about 10^8 molecules of plasmid DNA 10 h after immunization, while 24 h after immunization the number of plasmids decreased significantly. The most sensitive and specific method, PCR, using as a matrix DNA isolated from the injection site at different times after injection and oligonucleotides corresponding to the pSVK3-ENS1 plasmid injected, confirmed the presence of at least 10^8 molecules of plasmid DNA at 10 h after injection and about 10^4 molecules at 24 h. At 48 h after injection, all attempts at plasmid detection were unsuccessful. To estimate the amounts of plasmids isolated from the muscle tissue of immunized mice, quantities of PCR products were compared using serial 10-fold dilutions of the plasmid used as matrix. Taking into account that 100 µg of injected plasmid DNA corresponds to 10^{13} molecules, we can estimate the fraction remaining 10 h after plasmid injection as 0.001% and 24 h after injection as 0.0000001%. The data obtained indicate the low stability of plasmid DNA not only *in vitro,* but also *in vivo.*

In addition to plasmid instability, rearrangements of exogenous DnA in eukaryotic cells are possible. Already 48 h after transfection of eukaryotic cells, mutations appear in plasmid DNA (MacGregor et al., 1987), mostly in cell lines with reduced ability to repair (Finn et al., 1989).

Recombinant plasmids based on eukaryotic expression vectors pSVK3, pcDNAI, and pREP9-M2 were injected into 3 transfected monolayer cultures of human kidney RH, canine MDCK, and porcine SPEV cells for analysis of genetic rearrangements of plasmid DNA at the late stages of transfection. Transfection levels were assessed using lipofectin and DOTAP cationic lipid or electroporation under selective conditions in the presence of appropriate antibiotics, the resistance genes to which are encoded by the analyzed plasmids. Addition of antibiotics to the culture media allowed only transfected cells to be selected. It turned out that the level of cell culture transfection did not exceed 10-5, which was consistent with the results described earlier (Yates et al., 1985). At various time intervals after transfection, plasmids were isolated from eukaryotic cells by alkaline denaturation (Maniatis et al., 1984), based on the high copy number of small episomes compared to the high molecular weight genome, recovered by transformation of competent bacterial *Escherichia coli* cells, and compared with the original plasmid by restriction analysis (Fig. 8). For recombinant plasmids based on the eukaryotic expression vector pSVK3, the identity of injected and recovered plasmid DNA from eukaryotic cells or mouse organs was shown. For derivatives of the pcDNAI vector, genetic rearrangements were detected in some of the plasmids recovered from transfected eukaryotic cells. The maximum mutation frequency was detected for plasmids based on the pREP9 vector. At 4 weeks after transfection, which corresponds to 10 self-duplications of RH and MDCK cell cultures and 20 for SPEV cells, all recovered plasmids had rearrangements (Fig. 8). Mutations could occur randomly in all plasmid sites with different frequencies, but selection of transfected eukaryotic cells in the presence of neomycin and bacterial cells in the presence of ampicillin led to the identification of plasmids with wild-type antibiotic resistance genes. At the same time, the cloned viral genes were significantly altered. Deletions were the most numerous plasmid mutations in eukaryotic cells. Accumulation of shortened forms of plasmids has also been shown after transfection of eukaryotic cells with low repair capacity (Powell et al., 1993). The findings suggest that any plasmid fragment can be altered or deleted during replication in eukaryotic cells without selection for the corresponding gene product. Consequently, long-term continuous synthesis of the antigen as a result of injections of recombinant DnA without selection of transfected cells with the original plasmids is unlikely.

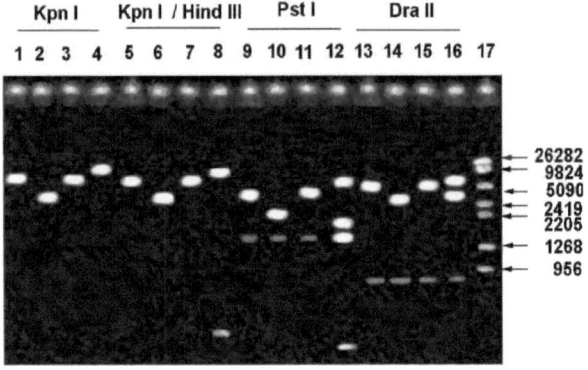

Figure 8. Results of restriction analysis of plasmids recovered from transfected human RH kidney cells (lanes 1, 5, 9, 13), pig SPEV (lanes 2, 6, 10, 14), dog MDCK (lanes 3, 7, 11, 15), and the original pREP9-M2 plasmid used for transfection (lanes 4, 8, 12, 16). Restriction endonucleases for plasmid hydrolysis are indicated at the top.

After DNA enters cells, some of it penetrates into nuclei through pores in nuclear membranes. This energy-dependent process does not depend on soluble cytoplasmic protein factors (Dowty et al., 1995). Most plasmids in eukaryotic cells remain in an extrachromosomal state (Cohen, 1993; Zhu et al., 1993; Xiong et al., 1997). However, as a result of exogenous DNA penetration into host cell nuclei, malignant transformation is possible through insertion of an active oncogene, activation of a cellular protooncogene, or insertional deactivation of a suppressor gene. Thus, after intramuscular injection, plasmid DNA was detected by PCR both in the total preparation and in chromosomal DNA purified from low-molecular-weight plasmids using gel electrophoresis. The integration of plasmids with DNA of differentiated or slowly dividing vertebrate cells occurs with frequencies 1000 times lower than the frequency of spontaneous mutagenesis or does not occur at all (Nichols et al., 1995), while cells with high reproductive activity are characterized by an increased probability of integration of replicating plasmids into the genome (Xiong et al., 1997). It has been shown that in the presence of an antibiotic resistance gene in the recombinant plasmid from some human cell lines resistant to this antibiotic and from all rodent lines studied, obtained by transfection with plasmid DNA, it is not possible to isolate plasmid DNA (Yates et al., 1985), which indicates the possible integration of the resistance gene into the host genome. Plasmids undetectable by hybridization several weeks after transfection with positive PCR results may also indicate incorporation (Zhu et al., 1993). Integration of plasmid DNA during long-term persistence into genomes of rapidly dividing B-lymphocytes, splenocytes and macrophages with a frequency of $D10^{-7}$ has now been proven (Liljeqvist and Stahl, 1999). It should be noted that the probability of plasmid integration increased with increasing eukaryotic DNA replication rate in rapidly dividing cells (Xiong et al., 1997).

At least 10 μg of DNA from transfected cells must be analyzed by Southern hybridization (Maniatis et al., 1984) to detect plasmid integration into a cellular genome of approximately 3×10^9 np. Since the estimated frequency of incorporation is significantly less than 1 plasmid per genome, the sensitivity level of hybridization methods is insufficient for detection. Therefore, a combination of PCR with primers corresponding to repetitive sequences of the eukaryotic genome (Alu repeats, $(AC)_6$, and T16) (Ilyin and Georgiev, 1982; Jurka and Smith, 1988; Moreau et al., 1982, respectively) and plasmid was used for amplification of certain genome regions followed by Southern hybridization with a radioactively labeled plasmid fragment.

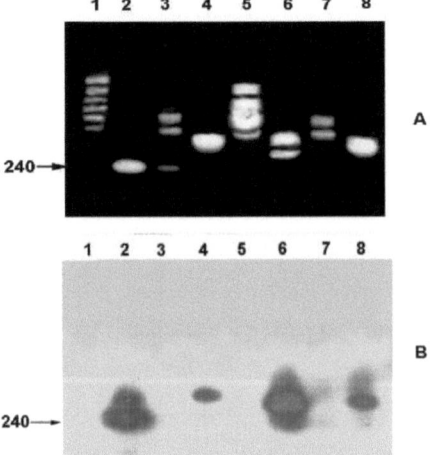

Fig. 9. Analysis of PCR products with primers corresponding to the Alu repeats of the eukaryotic genome and plasmid fragment.

A. Electrophoregram of PCR products using 2 matrices - initial plasmid pREP9-M2 and DNA from control untransfected ETP cells (lanes 1-4) or total DNA from ETP cells 5 months after transfection with plasmid pREP9-M2 (lanes 5-8). The following primers were used: Alu-consensus oligonucleotide (lanes 1, 5), virus-specific primers N1 and N2 (lanes 2, 6), Alu and N1 (lanes 3, 7), Alu and N2 (lanes 4, 8).

B. Results of Southern hybridization of amplicons with a radioactively labeled plasmid fragment corresponding to the cloned viral gene. Track numbers correspond to part A. The arrow on the left indicates the position of the 240 nb PCR product.

The observed differences in PCR products with a hybrid pair of primers corresponding to eukaryotic genome repeats and recombinant plasmid for the original plasmid and DNA from transfected cells (Fig. 9A and B) may indicate the possible integration of plasmid DNA into the genome of host cells.

Thus, instability, multiple mutations, and the possibility of plasmids being inserted into cellular chromosomes may reduce the protective effect of gene immunization. It should be noted that the frequency of genomic DNA rearrangements was significantly lower than that of extrachromosomal plasmid mutations (Fig. 8-9). This could be due to the protection of cellular DNA by chromatin proteins against nucleases. Eukaryotic expression vectors integrating into specific regions of the cellular genome are currently lacking (Calos, 1996). Creation of such vectors for directed integration of exogenous DnA into functionally inert regions of cellular DnA will probably lead to a decrease in rearrangements of exogenous DnA without damaging the genetic apparatus of the host cell and without elimination of unreplicating plasmids.

2.1.1. Study of VCE gene expression in eukaryotic cells

When purified recombinant DnA is introduced into eukaryotic cells, prolonged persistence of plasmids in nuclei can lead to continuous expression of cloned viral genes and, consequently, constant induction of a protective immune response. Despite the instability of plasmids in eukaryotic cells and possible integration into chromosomes occurring at very low frequencies, transcription of cloned viral genes by DNA-dependent RNA polymerase II occurs after some recombinant plasmids penetrate into eukaryotic cell nuclei. The promoters of the pre-early cytomegalovirus (CMV) and Raus sarcoma virus (RSV) genes are considered to be the strongest promoters currently known. The potency of other known oncogenic virus (SV40) promoters as well as cellular gene promoters, particularly mouse glucocorticoid, keratinocyte K17 or Langerhans cell CD11b promoters, is less than 10% of the strength of CMV or RSV promoters.

The RNA of viral genes obtained as a result of transcription in cell nuclei is translated on ribosomes of the cell to form full-length viral proteins. Synthesis and presentation of foreign proteins

from host cells are similar to viral infection. But with qualitative similarities, significant quantitative differences are observed. Gene immunization results in antigen amounts from 10-12 g/ml to 10-9 g/ml (Tighea et al., 1998) significantly less than viral infection, and synthesis takes longer (in skeletal muscle, up to 6 months) (Raz et al., 1994; Bot et al., 1996; Taubes, 1997).

Expression of nonstructural NS1 and NS3 VKE genes in transplanted cells 24 and 72 h after transfection with pSVK3-ENS1 and pcDNAI-NS3 plasmids using

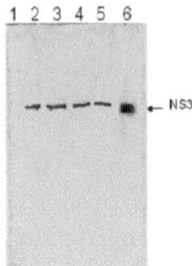

1 2 3 4 5 6

← NS3

DOTAP cationic lipid or electroporation was shown by immunoblotting with specific monoclonal antibodies (Figure 10).

Fig. 10. Analysis of NS3 gene expression of VKE in transfected SPEV cells. Results of immunoblotting with monoclonal antibodies to NS3 protein. Lane 1 - proteins of control uninfected cells, lanes 2-5 - proteins from transfected cells after 24 h (lanes 2 and 4) and 72 h after injection of pcDNAI-NS3 plasmid DNA (lanes 3 and 5). Transfection was performed using DOTAP cationic lipid (lanes 2 and 3) and by electroporation (lanes 4 and 5). Track 6 - Proteins of VCE-infected SPEV cells 36 h after infection.

96 h after transfection under non-selective conditions, the level of VCE gene expression became below the sensitivity limit of enzyme immunoassay using monoclonal antibodies and mouse anti-immunoglobulin antibody conjugate with alkaline phosphatase. This could probably be the result of plasmid degradation or mutations in dividing eukaryotic cells. Attempts to detect VKE antigens in mouse tissue homogenates after intramuscular and intradermal injections, as well as after ballistic transfection with plasmid DNA pSVK3-ENS1 and pcDNAI-NS3 by immunoassay using poly- or monoclonal antibodies to E, NS1 and NS3 VKE proteins were not successful. This was probably due to the low level of transfection, not

exceeding 10-5 for cell cultures, and the limit of sensitivity of the immunoassay being 10-9 d (Matveev et al. , 1989).

After translation, the viral proteins synthesized in the cytosol are proteolytically degraded to peptides, which are transported to the endoplasmic reticulum. Here, the peptides interact with Major Histocompatibility Complex (MHC1) molecules and are then transported to the cell surface for recognition by CD8+ T-helpers. In turn, Th lymphocytes orchestrate an immune response by stimulating antibody production by B cells, clonal expansion of cytotoxic lymphocytes, and activating macrophage killer cells (Sartakova and Konenkov, 1997).

The humoral immune response after administration of DNA vaccines is weak or not detectable at all because of the small amounts of antigens produced, resulting in inadequate stimulation of B-cells. CD4+ T-helper cells are known to divide into populations according to the cytokines secreted. After antigenic stimulation, Th1 cells synthesize interleukin 2 (IL-2) and interferon-D, whereas 'Th2 cells produce the interleukins IL-4, IL-5, IL-6 and IL-10. Two signals are required for induction of antigen-specific cytotoxic T lymphocytes: 1) recognition of an MHC1-bound peptide on the cell surface; 2) a nonspecific costimulatory signal, which requires specialized antigen-presenting cells (Tighea et al., 1998). The Th1 immune response stimulates macrophage activation to inactivate intracellular pathogens, promotes delayed-type hypersensitivity, and enhances the synthesis of IgG2a and IgG3 isotypes of antibodies (Tighea et al., 1998). DNA vaccination has been found to result in a type 1 (Th1) T-helper response. This immune response develops even in newborn animals, despite the deficiency and immaturity of cytotoxic CD8 T-lymphocytes, natural killer cells and macrophages in the early stages of life (Martinez et al., 1997). The developing cellular immune response leads to the elimination of intracellular microorganisms and viruses. After primary immunization with protein followed by secondary vaccination with DNA, a Th1 response is formed. If the DNA is injected first and then the protein, the Th1 response persists. Consequently, the immune response induced by DNA vaccination is dominant (Debabov, 1997).

In spite of non-dectable VEE antigens in animal tissues, specific antibodies were detected in the blood of immunized mice after injections of recombinant plasmids. A comparison of antibody titers against structural glycoprotein E of VSE after injection of plasmid pSVK3-ENS1 or inactivated protein vaccines is shown in Table 2. It should be noted that inactivated protein vaccines contain 0.75-4.5 µg of E VSE protein in single doses (Table 1). Differences in the ranges of antibody titers after immunization of mice with inactivated vaccine Encevir (Microgen, Tomsk) and FSME-IMMUN (Baxter, Austria), as well as low antibody titers after DNA vaccines directly correlate with the content of injected E VSE antigen (Tables 1 and 2). Therefore, the humoral immune response induced by traditional vaccines was stronger compared to gene immunization. However, the immune response after DNA injection is more durable compared to inactivated vaccines (Chen et al., 1999). Gene immunization induces a predominantly cellular immune response through the Th1 pathway that provides protection against viral infections (Martinez et al., 1997; Debabov, 1997; Sartakova and Konenkov, 1997).

Table 2. Determination of antibodies to VSE proteins in the sera of mice after immunization with different vaccines.

Types of vaccines against VEE	Protein antibody titers WCE
Inactivated purified vaccine produced by Encevir (Microgen, Tomsk)	1:600 - 1:900
Inactivated purified vaccine FSME-IMMUN (Baxter, Austria)	1:300 - 1:600
Native glycoprotein NS1 (Pressman et al., 1993)	1:100.000
Recombinant NS1 protein (Pressman et al., 1993)	1:100.000 - 1:10.000.000

Bacteria transformed with pUR290(NS1)₂ plasmid	1:100 - 1:500
Plasmid DNA pSVK3-ENS1, pSVK3-E and pSVK3-prME	1:10 - 1:100
Full-length VKE RNAs	1:20 - 1:40

Antibodies to the nonstructural proteins NS1 and NS3 of VKE with average titers of 1:100 were detected by enzyme immunoassay in blood sera of mice immunized with recombinant DNA pSVK3-ENS1 and pcDNAI-NS3, respectively. Antibodies to the nonstructural proteins NS1 and NS3 of VCE in the blood of mice after gene immunization were also recorded by immunoblotting with monoclonal antibodies. Antibodies to linear epitopes of the NS1 VKE protein with titers of 1:50 were detected in 3 of 15 mice after pSVK3-ENS1 DNA injections, and only one of 15 sera showed antibodies to the NS3 protein after pcDNAI-NS3 plasmid injection. It should be noted that an antigen-specific, dose-dependent cellular immune response also does not develop in every organism after gene immunization (e.g., only 11 of 17 healthy volunteers after DNA vaccination against malaria) (Brower, 1998). Such antibodies were absent in the sera of intact animals and mice immunized with pSVK3 and pcDNA vector DNA and 1000-fold diluted inactivated protein vaccines. It should be emphasized that immunization with more than 100-fold diluted inactivated protein vaccines did not induce the development of a humoral immune response, whereas gene immunization, leading to the synthesis of about 10-12 g of viral protein (Taubes, 1997), induced the formation of detectable amounts of antibodies (Table 2). Consequently, the formation of viral antigens in transfected and infected cells has advantages over the introduction of foreign proteins (Sartakova and Konenkov, 1997). A weak humoral immune response (Phillpotts et al., 1996) or lack of detectable amounts of specific antibodies (Hosie et al., 1998) are characteristic of DNA immunization. It has been suggested that low antibody titers after intramuscular gene immunization may be due to the absence of antigen-presenting cells in the muscle (Raz et al., 1994). However, intradermal injections of plasmids and ballistic transfection also did not significantly increase specific antibody titers despite the abundance of antigen-presenting cells in the skin (Raz et al., 1994). This may be explained by the low efficiency of plasmid DNA capture by skin cells compared to myocytes.

In addition, antibodies obtained by immunizing mice with the plasmid pSVK3-ENS1 did not have virus-neutralizing properties, despite the presence of polyclonal antibodies to the virion envelope protein E (Table 2). Similar results about the absence of neutralizing antibodies were obtained for other flavivirus species (Phillpotts et al., 1996).

Thus, despite low levels of eukaryotic cell transfection and expression of cloned viral genes, administration of recombinant plasmids pSVK3-ENS1 and pcDNAI-NS3 to mice resulted in the appearance of antibodies to VCE proteins. Consequently, plasmid instability does not prevent the development of humoral immunity. Apparently, trace amounts of viral antigens synthesized over several days are sufficient for the induction of protective immunity.

As a result of infection of mice after intramuscular immunization with 4 recombinant plasmids with lethal doses of homologous VKE strain, the minimum number of surviving animals was recorded for the groups immunized with recombinant plasmid DNA pcDNAI-NS3 (60+16.3), pSVK3 or pcDNAI vectors (42.9+20.2%) and for the intact group (61.9+10.9%) (Figure 11).

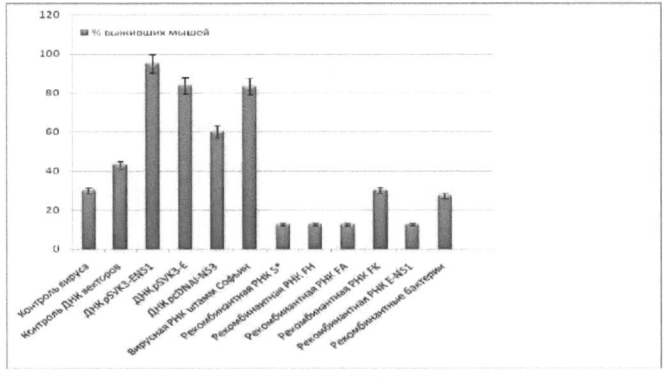

The following signs of tick-borne encephalitis in mice were observed. On the 9th day after infection some mice were agitated, on the 10th day the animals showed characteristic signs of tick-borne encephalitis - lethargy, tremor, refusal of food, limb paralysis. The death of mice usually occurred on days 10-16 after infection. Differences between control groups of intact and vector-vaccinated animals and mice immunized with pcDNAI-NS3 plasmid were not significant. The absence of a protective effect in the presence of antibodies directed to the VKE NS3 protein after immunization of mice with pcDNAI-NS3 DNA is probably explained by the inaccessibility of the intracellular nonstructural viral protein NS3 to antibodies and immune system cells. Gene immunization with recombinant plasmids containing the C, NS1-NS2A, NS3, and NS5 genes of Japanese encephalitis virus also does not provide protection against infection with a homologous strain of the virus (Chen et al., 1999). Consequently, the phenomenon of replicase-mediated resistance (Carr and Zaitlin, 1993) has not been found for VEE as for other animal viruses.

The highest survival rate of mice after immunization with pSVK3-ENS1 plasmid DNA was statistically significantly ($p<0.05$) different from that of the control groups (Fig. 11). Animals immunized with purified plasmid pSVK3-ENS1 remained healthy during the whole period of observation - 30 days, activity was moderate and stable without signs of agitation or lethargy, loss of appetite was not noted either. However, with increasing doses of VCE, mortality was also observed among immunized animals. The number of surviving animals decreased with increasing doses of the virus (Table 3), which was nevertheless significantly different from mortality among intact animals ($p<0.05$). The combination of low titers of antibodies to E and NS1 VSE proteins in mice after gene immunization with pSVK3-ENS1 plasmid (Table 2) and a marked protective response (Fig. 11) could be due to a cellular immune response (Debabov, 1997).

Table 3: Dependence of the protective effect of intramuscular immunization with plasmid DNA pSVK3-ENS1 on the dose of VCE (homologous strain Sofjin).

Dose of VCE (in LD50)	10^2 LD50	10^4 LD50	10^5 LD50
Proportion of surviving mice immunized with pSVK3-ENS1 plasmid	95+5%	91,7+8,3%	85,7+14,3%

DNA vaccination is known to protect experimental animals against infectious diseases even without the induction of detectable amounts of specific antibodies (Hosie et al., 1998).

In the group of animals immunized intramuscularly with pSVK3-E plasmid DNA, 84.7+10.4% of animals survived after infection with the homologous Sofjin VSE strain (Fig. 11). After infection with the virus, mice immunized with pSVK3-prME plasmid DNA survived 66.7+15.7% of the animals, which was less than the relative number of surviving mice after immunization with pSVK3-ENS1 DNA. Similar results of vaccination with recombinant plasmid with cloned prM and E genes were obtained for St. Louis virus belonging to the family *Flaviviridae* (Phillpotts et al., 1996). The smaller protective effect of pSVK3-E and pSVK3-prME plasmids compared with pSVK3-ENS1 DNA may have been due to the localization of E and prM proteins on the virion surface and within infected cells, whereas the nonstructural glycoprotein NS1 is expressed on the cell surface and secreted from infected cells in homo- and heterodimer forms (Schlesinger et al., 1985). Consequently, the presence of virion surface protein genes in plasmids caused a lower protective effect compared to viral genes whose products are on the surface of infected cells (Phillpotts et al., 1996; Schmaljohn et al., 1997; Lin et al., 1998). The high level of protection against Japanese encephalitis virus infection by recombinant E-gene plasmids in the absence of the protective effect of cloned NS1-NS2A genes (Chen et al., 1999) was probably the result of incomplete cleavage between NS1 and NS2A proteins, which excluded surface localization of the nonstructural glycoprotein

NS1 dimer on plasma membranes of transfected cells and contact with the host immune system. DNA immunization with a plasmid containing the individual NS1 gene of the same Japanese encephalitis virus protected animals against lethal doses of the homologous virus strain (Lin et al., 1998). In addition, there is ample evidence for protection against flavivirus infection when the NS1 gene is expressed in various heterologous systems (for references, see Pressman et al., 1993; Timofeev et al., 1998). The greatest protective effect of plasmids with the cloned NS1 gene of flaviviruses seems to be due to the need to eliminate infected cells rather than only extracellular viral particles. Consequently, cellular immunity is required to eliminate viral infection.

Thus, the combination of glycoproteins E and NS1 in the transfected cells provided the greatest protective effect against infection with the homologous VEE strain, while injections of pSVK3-E and pSVK3-prME plasmid DNA caused less protection against the virus. Injection of pcDNAI-NS3 DNA containing the nonstructural NS3 VSE gene did not result in protection of animals against VSE (Fig. 11).

It is possible to clone not full-length viral genes but only their fragments encoding immunogenic epitopes 9-11 a.s. When cloned in various vector systems, such "minigens" proved capable of inducing cytotoxic T-lyphocytes similar in affinity and cytokine secretion to those induced by viral infection. However, immunization with purified plasmid DNA containing short fragments of viral genes encoding antigenic determinants does not result in protection against lethal viral infection. "Minigenes" have protective properties only as part of recombinant smallpox vaccine viruses (Rodriguez et al., 1998). Induction of the immune response by "minigenes" cloned in eukaryotic expression vectors can be significantly enhanced by covalent attachment of ubiquitin to protein fragments (Xiang et al., 2000). It is known that most of the peptides that bind to the major histocompatibility complex type 1 MHC1 for induction of cytotoxic T lymphocytes are formed in proteosomes. Proteins are directed to these organelles by covalent attachment of many copies of the cellular protein ubiquitin. Therefore, foreign proteins after ubiquitin attachment are more rapidly degraded to peptides in cellular proteosomes and are more efficiently presented to the immune system and, consequently, induce an immune response (Xiang et al., 2000).

Thus, despite their cheapness, storage stability, and induction of cellular and humoral immunity, current DNA vaccine candidates have significant drawbacks. Clearly, the ongoing clinical trials of such gene vaccines in the United States are premature. Antibodies directed to DnA are capable of inducing autoimmune diseases. Instability and genetic rearrangements of recombinant DnA probably disrupt the expression of cloned viral genes. The incorporation of recombinant DNA into cellular chromosomes occurs randomly and can cause serious genetic disorders. Since the genomes of all eukaryotes are characterized by the presence of heterochromatin consisting of highly repetitive fractions and moderate repeats, in which genes are almost absent, the design of vectors for directed episome integration into genetically inert heterochromatin regions would increase the stability and safety of DNA vaccines. Persistent expression of viral genes can lead to tolerance to the pathogen or other negative allergic reactions (Bot et al., 1996). Since DNA vaccines are supposed to be used to prevent infectious diseases in healthy children, further thorough testing of their safety is necessary.

Promising candidates for DNA vaccines have been obtained for a number of flaviviruses: VEE (Schmaljohn et al., 1997), Japanese encephalitis virus, Dengue and yellow fever viruses, and St. Louis virus (for references, see Chen et al., 1999).

2.1.2. RNA immunization

RNA immunization reduces the risk of genomic rearrangements while preserving the benefits of presenting the antigen "from within" the transfected cells. Various injectable and noninvasive methods are used to deliver RNA into cells, including ballistic transfection of animal skin with mRNA-coated gold particles (Liljeqvist and Stahl, 1999).

To obtain recombinant RNA, an *Escherichia coli* BL21 strain containing a cloned T7 phage RNA polymerase gene was transfected with plasmids including both a full-length DNA copy of the VKE genome (Sofjin strain) and individual E, NS1, and NS3 genes under control of the T7 promoter. At various times after isopropylthiogalactoside (IPTG) induction of the T7 phage DNA-dependent RNA polymerase promoter followed by *in vivo* intracellular transcription, recombinant VKE RNA was isolated from bacterial cells and intramuscularly immunized into BALB/c mice. The protective effect was detected only after administration of full-length genomic RNA isolated from brain suspensions of mice infected with a homologous strain of Sofjin VKE, but not recombinant genomic RNA S*, FH, FA, FK with different in length, structure, and degree of polyadenylation 3'-untranslated regions (3'UTR) or genome fragments containing genes of surface antigens E and NS1 (Fig. 11) or the nonstructural protein gene NS3. The construction of recombinant and chimeric RNA-containing viruses does not ensure the homogeneity of genomic RNA quasispecies due to replication errors during rapid viral reproduction and the absence of RNA repair systems in the host cells, nor does it rule out recombination with endogenous flaviviruses and the possibility of selection of pathogenic variants. Only recombinant attenuated flaviviruses obtained by co-transfection of cell cultures with several plasmid DNAs with cloned genome fragments can ensure relative safety. Such approaches to vaccine creation are currently being developed by Safari Pasteur (USA).

2.2. Recombinant bacteria

Recombinant bacteria administered to mucosal membranes are a promising area of infectious disease prevention. The advantages of mucosal vaccines are the ease of administration without a syringe and the induction of not only systemic but also local immunity at the entrance gate of respiratory, intestinal and urogenital infections (Gendon, 1999). Endogenous and exogenous plasmids in bacterial cells are more stable than in eukaryotic cells. The widespread exchange of genetic information among prokaryotes leads to the modular organization of plasmids isolated from natural sources (O'Sullivan and Klaenhammer, 1993).

Nonpathogenic bacteria that form colonies on mucous membranes are capable of expressing foreign genes. Among Gram-negative bacteria, *Escherichia coli, Salmonella spp., Shigella flexneri, Yersinia enterocolitica* and *Bordetella pertussis are* the most studied as producers of foreign proteins (Liljeqvist and Stahl, 1999). *Escherichia coli is a* natural inhabitant of the human gut, hence elimination of these bacteria by antibodies and cytotoxic T cells is unlikely. However, despite numerous studies on heterologous gene expression, surface localization and immunogenicity of the antigens they encode, *E. coli* is considered an experimental delivery system and is not considered a live vaccine, since natural strains are conditionally pathogenic and unable to maintain replication of foreign DNA due to restriction and modification enzymes, and laboratory attenuated strains are unable to survive in animals and humans.

Salmonella typhi forms colonies on the intestinal mucosa and multiplies in associated lymphoid tissue, later spreading to the liver and spleen, leading to the serious pathology known as typhoid fever. All clinical and field trials of Salmonella are conducted using attenuated strains. While pathogenic strains of *Salmonella typhimurium* kill the M cells of peyer's plaques when they penetrate and cannot penetrate the underlying mucosal layers, vaccine attenuated strains leave the M and dendritic cells viable, ensuring presentation of the antigen to the mucosal immune system. As intracellular pathogens, live salmonellae induce cellular immunity directed toward a heterologous protein. The presence of IgG1 and IgG2 immunoglobulins indicates a Th1 and Th2 type immune response, which is an advantage of recombinant intracellular bacteria over extracellular bacteria as vaccines (Corthesy-Theulaz et al., 1998). A disadvantage of recombinant *S. typhimurium* cells is the risk of side effects due to potential reversion to virulent wild strains in people with immunopathologies. Clinical trials of recombinant salmonellae in humans have not shown positive results. Therefore, recombinant *Salmonella* bacteria are currently used to study the expression of foreign genes, but not as live vaccines (Karpenko et al., 2000).

Among Gram-positive bacteria, attenuated strains of Mycobacterium BCG (bacille Calmette-Guerin) and *Staphylococcus aureus* were initially used to express heterologous genes. Mycobacteria are intracellular pathogens that induce cellular and humoral immunity. Live vaccines based on Gram-positive bacteria are in human clinical trials. Nonpathogenic commensal bacteria and lactic acid bacteria used in the food industry and providing stable expression of foreign genes are being investigated. (O'Sullivan and Klaenhammer, 1993; Pouwels et al. , 1996). For such non-pathogenic bacteria, there is no risk of reversion to the wild-type virulent phenotype and elimination of the resulting recombinants by an induced immune response (Liljeqvist and Stahl, 1999).

To present a heterologous antigen to the host immune system, its localization on the surface of bacterial cells is desirable. Currently, gene expression systems have been developed for cytoplasmic and secreted proteins of Gram-negative and Gram-positive bacteria. Surface localization of model antigens has been shown by inserting foreign genes into genes of outer membrane proteins, lipoproteins, or cell appendix proteins (Liljeqvist and Stahl, 1999). Some surface expression systems involve sequential stages of translocation and "anchoring" of the protein on the surface. For example, the protease IgA *of Neisseria gonorrhoeae*, when embedded in the membrane, forms a pore through which the antigen fused to it is translocated. Pullulanase *of Klebsiella pneumoniae* is found on the bacterial surface temporarily when secreted into the culture medium. In Gram-negative bacteria, cell walls are surrounded by an outer membrane whose membrane lipopolysaccharides are natural adjuvants for the polypeptides on the surface.

Localization of foreign proteins on the surface of recombinant bacteria is also an obvious advantage for Gram-positive bacteria (Nguyen et al., 1995). The mechanisms of surface protein "anchoring" are common to all Gram-positive bacteria. The C-terminal region of such proteins consists of a region of charged repeating amino acid residues interacting with the cell wall peptidoglycan, a highly conserved cleavage site by proteolytic enzymes LPXTG, a hydrophobic transmembrane fragment 15-20 a.s. long and a hydrophilic region. After proteolytic cleavage between the threonine and glycine residues of the LPXTG motif, the surface protein covalently attaches to the cell wall (Liljeqvist and Stahl, 1999).

Currently, most studies are devoted to the induction of various types of immunity after the introduction of recombinant bacteria. Intracellular localization of heterologous proteins results in the impossibility of inducing an immune response, while mucosal secretion from bacteria causes rapid elimination of the antigen from the body. Limited infection with attenuated strains of bacteria, as well as natural infection with pathogenic strains, results in a strong and prolonged immune response in the host organism. Since attenuated bacteria are capable of surviving in higher organisms for some time, this leads to an extended duration of the immune response. Thus, attenuated pathogenic bacteria have advantages over mucosal inhabitants for the induction of immunity. Immunization with recombinant *Escherichia coli* cells containing viral antigens in the periplasmic space resulted in antibody formation in mice (Leclerc et al., 1990). Other bacterial surface components, such as lipopolysaccharides, are natural adjuvants of Gram-negative bacteria for surface polypeptides. Gram-positive lactic acid bacteria cells are also good adjuvants (Pouwels et al., 1996; Locht, 2000). The surface lipopolysaccharides of microorganisms and oligonucleotides are synergistic, leading to the release of cytokines and activation of mammalian immunized macrophages (Sparwasser et al., 1997). Specific antibodies are usually undetectable in intracellular localization of antigens. Oral administration of antigens in combination with probiotic bacteria, induces a local mucosal immune response through the type 2 T-helper pathway, which may be enhanced by subsequent intradermal administration of the antigen (Chin et al., 2000).

Recombinant bacteria can provide only partial protection against infection (Gendon, 1999). For example, intranasal administration of *Lactococcus lactis, which* forms tetanus toxin, provides 75% protection in mice. Recombinant *Salmonella typhimurium cells* expressing the *Helicobacter pylori* urease gene protected only 60% of animals from subsequent infection (Locht, 2000).

Recombinant bacteria are the cheapest way to obtain vaccines, since they are capable of reproduction and do not require purified antigen isolation. Recombinant plasmids in bacteria are more stable than in eukaryotic cells, and the risk of integrating foreign DNA into the prokaryotic genome is not dangerous for the immunized organism. The expression of heterologous genes in bacterial cells induces local and systemic immunity. A significant disadvantage of such mucosal vaccines is the presentation of protein antigens "from outside" and hence the preferential formation of antibodies. The weak cytotoxic immune response does not suppress intracellular viral, bacterial or protozoal infections. The advantage of injecting recombinant bacteria into the nasopharyngeal mucosa compared to the digestive tract is the absence of degradation of protein antigens in the stomach prior to contact with immune system cells.

Since the introduction of purified plasmid DNA pSVK3-ENS1 provided the highest level of protection against VSE infection (Fig. 11), the construction of recombinant bacteria expressing the NS1 VSE gene would allow us to compare the effectiveness of different ways of presenting this antigen.

It is known that introduction of new bacteria to mucous membranes meets resistance of endogenous inhabitants. Therefore, an *ex vivo* approach of plasmid transformation of natural bacterial strains isolated from the nasopharyngeal mucosa of linear mice followed by intranasal administration of recombinant bacteria to animals was proposed. Transformation of bacterial cells of various families is performed by a variety of methods, the most universal of which is electroporation. Introduction of plasmid DNA pUR290(NS1)$_2$ with 0-lactamase (ampicillinase) and NS1 VCE genes (5 pulses of 30 ms at 300 V) gave rise to ampicillin-resistant cell clones. Extraction of plasmid DNA from clones of transformed cells for 10 consecutive passages followed by restriction analysis proved the identity of the original DNA used for electroporation and the isolated plasmids. Consequently, plasmid pUR290(NS1)$_2$ is stable in the bacterial strains studied. It turned out that the stability of exogenous DNA in prokaryotic cells is significantly higher than in eukaryotic cells.

Synthesis of the NS1 VKE protein in transformed bacterial cells after addition of isopropylthiogalactoside (IPTG) was shown by immunoblotting with specific monoclonal antibodies (Fig. 12). Without prior induction of the lac promoter, the expression level of the viral NS1 gene was below the sensitivity limit of immunoblotting with monoclonal antibodies to the VSE NS1 protein. The 39 kDa molecular weight of the recombinant NS1 protein determined by electrophoresis in SDS-PAAG was consistent with that expected theoretically (Mandl et al., 1989; Pletnev et al., 1990). *The* presence of the NS1 VKE protein was shown in both bacterial cells and in the culture fluid (Fig. 12 A and B). The viral protein was detected predominantly in the precipitate after centrifugation at 14,000 g. Because the

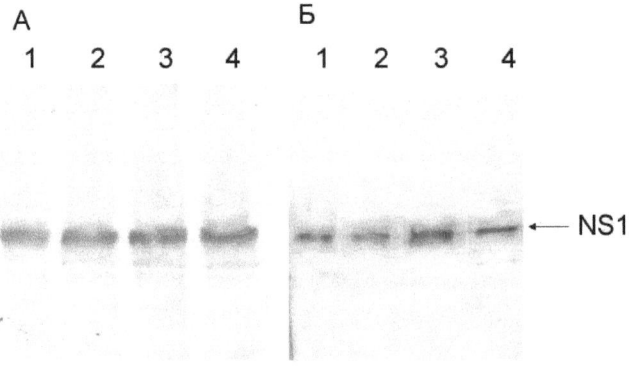

nonstructural glycoprotein NS1 is known to reside on surface membranes and is secreted from

mammalian and insect cells (Schlesinger et al., 1986), its localization in bacterial cells may be similar. Prokaryotes are characterized by the absence of intracellular lipid membranes, so the localization of the viral antigen on the plasma membrane of cells cannot be ruled out. However, given the probability of the formation of insoluble "inclusion bodies" in the cytoplasm of bacterial progenitors and the difference in the signal sequences required for protein secretion from bacterial and eukaryotic cells, the presence of the NS1 protein in the culture fluid can be explained by the destruction of recombinant bacteria.

Fig.12. Results of immunoblotting of recombinant bacterial proteins with monoclonal antibodies to the native glycoprotein NS1 of VKE.
A - Cell proteins; B - culture fluid proteins. Lanes 1-3 - proteins of recombinant bacteria, lane 4 - proteins of *E. coli*.

For taxonomic determination, recombinant bacteria isolated from mouse nasopharyngeal mucosa and transformed with pUR290(NS1)$_2$ plasmid were grown on LB medium. It turned out that they were immobile Gram-negative bacilli 5-20 μm long and 0.7-0.8 μm thick with the following features corresponding to Bergy's bacterial identifier (Bergy, 1980). The bacteria are facultative anaerobes, metabolism of tryptophan is accompanied by release of indole, urea is not used, glucose is digested heteroenzymatically, with positive reaction to "Methylrot," acidify Hiss medium with maltose, fructose and glucose, but not acidify with rhamnose, xylose, sucrose, mannitol, sorbitol, glycerol and gluconate; does not hydrolyze gelatin. Based on the above features, according to (Bergi, 1980), the transformed bacteria can be assigned to the family *Enterobacteriaceae* and genera *Edwardsiella* and *Shigella*. Obviously, the composition of nutrient media, mechanisms of plasmid replication and heterologous gene expression are common to various Gram-negative Enterobacteriaceae.

It is interesting to note that all the ampicillin-resistant bacterial strains studied were Gram-negative, which may be due to the following reasons. Introduction of plasmids through the thin cell wall of Gram-negative bacteria appears to be more effective compared to Gram-positive bacteria surrounded by a multilayer murein shell. Replication of recombinant plasmids with the ColE replication initiation site ori depends on DNA polymerases in Gram-negative bacteria and is hardly possible in Gram-positive prokaryotes. In addition, the molecular mechanisms of gene expression in Gram-positive bacteria differ significantly from Gram-negative cells, especially at the translation initiation stage, which could cause the lack of resistance to ampicillin in transformed Gram-positive commensals. It turned out that Gram-positive lactic acid bacteria, inhabitants of the nasopharyngeal mucosa of mice, are not cultured in LB nutrient medium. Therefore, the growth of recombinant bacteria on solid LB nutrient media with ampicillin resulted in the selection of only recombinant bacteria of the family *Enterobacteriaceae.*

To study the antigenicity and immunogenicity of the recombinant NS1 VCE protein, transformed Enterobacteriaceae were injected intranasally into mice

200 μl of overnight culture 15 times daily and antibodies in sera and mucosal wipes of mice were determined by immoblotting with the native glycoprotein NS1 of VSE from infected eukaryotic cells (Fig. 13). Antibodies were detected in sera at dilutions of 1:100 to 1:500. There were no antibodies directed to the NS1 VSE protein in

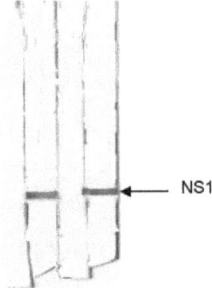

mucosal washes.

Fig.13. Detection of antibodies in blood sera of mice after intranasal immunization with recombinant bacteria presenting the NS1 VSE gene. Lanes 1, 3 - results of immunoblotting with proteins from control uninfected cells, lanes 2 and 4 - with proteins from VCE-infected eukaryotic cells. Lanes 1, 2 - immunoblotting with antibodies from mouse serum immunized with transformed *Edwardsiella* cells; 3, 4 - with mouse antibodies after intranasal immunization with recombinant *Shigella* bacteria.

Inactivated pathogens or individual proteins are known to penetrate poorly into mucosal cells and, therefore, are rapidly eliminated from the body before interacting with the nasopharyngeal immune system (Gendon, 1999). In this case, the bacterial cells serve as a mucosal-adhesive adjuvant, facilitating the contact of the heterologous protein with the mucosal cells and protecting the antigen from destruction. Perhaps, therefore, intranasal immunization of mice with recombinant bacteria results in the induction of a systemic humoral immune response in the absence of local immunity, or the latter is very weak.

After infection of mice with lethal doses of VEE, the proportion of deaths among control and immunized animals did not differ (Fig. 11). The absence of the protective effect of mucosal immunization against VEE may be due to the presence of antibodies to the NS1 protein of VEE and the absence of cellular immunity. The nonstructural NS1 glycoprotein is located on the surface of infected cells and is absent in virions. Therefore, it is possible that extracellular viral particles that do not interact with antibodies against the nonstructural NS1 protein caused the development of viral infection with fatal outcomes in experimental animals.

It should be noted that antibodies to the native BCE NS1 glycoprotein and its genetically engineered analogue did not protect animals against viral infection, despite the ability to bind complement (Pressman et al., 1993). The recombinant bacteria synthesized the viral protein NS1, which had the size and epitopes of the native glycoprotein, which after endocytosis was apparently cleaved in the antigen-presenting cells into peptides 10 to 20 a.s. long. Such products of proteolytic processing of protein antigens in complex with molecules of the MHC II major histocompatibility complex are known to be exposed to the immune system of the host. The induction of a predominantly humoral immune response does not provide elimination of infected cells, which requires a cellular immune response (Sartakova and Konenkov, 1997). In addition, the presence of antibodies to VCE proteins in blood sera and cerebrospinal fluids of patients with tick-borne encephalitis does not prevent the development of severe forms of the disease (Matveeva et al., 1995). Induction of cellular immunity occurs during viral infection and gene immunization. Apparently, differences in the presentation of endogenous and exogenous antigens are important for protective immunity.

A second possible reason for the lack of protection against VEE is the impossibility of preventing infectious diseases of the central nervous system by mucosal immunization due to the presence of the blood-brain barrier. It is possible that mucosal immunity prevents infections arising or occurring on the mucous membranes of the body, which include respiratory, intestinal and urogenital infections and does not belong to VEE.

A third reason for the lack of protective effect of mucosal immunization against VEE may be the fact that *ex vivo* transformed bacteria are unable to survive on mucous membranes due to the presence of endogenous bacteria. All our attempts to isolate ampicillin-resistant bacteria from mucous membrane wipes of immunized animals were unsuccessful, which could be due to inefficiency of wipes and the need for scrapings. The survival of bacteria in higher organisms is known to increase the duration of the immune response (Gendon, 1999; Liljeqvist and Stahl, 1999). Therefore, the presence of antibodies to the NS1 protein for a short period of time is not sufficient to protect mice against VCE.

Thus, induction of the humoral immune response to the nonstructural NS1 VSE protein by recombinant bacteria did not result in protection against infection, although introduction of purified plasmid pSVK3-ENS1 with cloned E and NS1 VSE genes provided a significant protective effect (Fig. 11).

When evaluating the efficacy of immunization with nonstructural BSE NS1 protein after immunization of mice with purified NS1 glycoprotein or the corresponding genetically engineered analog, recombinant bacteria expressing the BSE NS1 gene, pSVK3-ENS1 plasmid DNA, or full-length BSE RNA, both the amounts of NS1 antigen (Table 4) and how it was presented to the host's immune system differed. Comparison of antibody titers against the NS1 protein in the sera of immunized mice (Table 2) showed a dependence on the amount of antigen administered.

Table 4. Content of VCE antigens.

Types of vaccines against VEE	Number of viral antigens in the immunizing dose
Inactivated purified vaccines produced by Microgen (Tomsk) and Baxter (Vienna, Austria)	At least 10^{-6} g of protein E with a total of $(1-10) \times 10^{-3}$ g of protein
Purified NS1 protein	30×10^{-6} g of glycoprotein or recombinant NS1 protein
Bacteria transformed plasmid pUR290(NS1)$_2$	4×10^{-6} g NS1 protein
DNA vaccines	Below the sensitivity level of the immunoassay (about 10^{-12}-10^{-9} g protein E, NS1 or prM at the injection site (Tighea et al., 1998)
Full-length VKE RNAs	10^{-9}-10^{-8} g protein E in homogenates organs

The low content of nonstructural proteins in inactivated vaccines produced by Microgen (Tomsk) and Baxter (Austria) did not allow the recording of specific antibodies against the NS1 glycoprotein. Gene immunization resulted in the synthesis of approximately 10^{-12} g of viral antigen, so it induced weak humoral immunity (Tables 2 and 4). Injections of full-length VCE RNA also resulted in low levels of NS1 viral protein accumulation (approximately 10^{-8} g) as measured by enzyme immunoassay titration with specific monoclonal antibodies and hence low titers of specific antibodies (Tables 2 and 4). After induction of the lactose operon by IPTG, the NS1 protein content in *E.coli* cells is at least 20 mg in 1 L of culture fluid (Fig. 12, Table 4). An immunizing dose equal to 200 μL of stationary culture of recombinant bacteria corresponded to 4 μg of viral protein. Therefore, intranasal vaccination of mice with 200 μL of recombinant bacteria induced antibodies directed to the NS1 protein in sera with higher titers than after DNA and RNA immunizations (Table 2). The reduced humoral immune response after mucosal immunization with 4 μg of recombinant antigen compared to intramuscular administration of 30 μg of NS1 glycoprotein or recombinant protein is probably due to incomplete capture of viral protein by mucosal antigen-presenting cells. Consequently, the efficiency of antibody formation directly correlated with the amount of NS1 VCE antigen administered, regardless of the endogenous or exogenous mode of presentation to the immune system (Tables 2 and 4). However, the protective effect differed after different mode of administration of the VKE antigen (Fig. 11). After DNA immunization with the pSVK3-ENS1 plasmid, the number of surviving animals was 71.4100%, depending on the dose of virus for infection. However, administration of the native glycoprotein NS1, its genetically engineered analogue (Pressman et al., 1993) or recombinant bacteria expressing the VSE NS1 gene on mucous membranes did not provide protection against virus infection. It should be noted that the protective effect of immunization did not correlate with antibody titers directed to the nonstructural NS1 VSE protein (Fig. 11, Table 2). When antibody levels were high after immunization with native or genetically engineered NS1 protein (Pressman et al., 1993), as well as with recombinant bacteria, animal death due to VKE infection occurred. This could be due to a lack of cellular immunity despite the presence of antibodies to the NS1 protein of VKE. The nonstructural glycoprotein NS1 is found on the surface of infected cells but not in virions (Schlesinger et al., 1985; Monath, 1986). It is likely that extracellular virions that do not interact with antibodies against the NS1 protein lead to the death of experimental animals. It is known that exogenous antigens after penetration into cells and proteolytic processing to peptides 10-20 a.s. long form a complex with molecules of the major histocompatibility complex type II (MHC II), which is exhibited on the cell surface for contact with the host immune system (Sartakova and Konenkov, 1997). The induction of a predominantly humoral immune response does not ensure the elimination of infected cells, which requires cellular immunity. The presence of antibodies to VCE proteins in blood serum and cerebrospinal fluid of patients with tick-borne encephalitis also does not prevent the development of severe forms of the disease (Matveeva et al., 1995). Induction of cellular immunity occurs during viral infection as well as as as a result of DNA and RNA immunizations during which the antigen synthesized on cellular ribosomes is hydrolyzed to peptides of 9 a.o. and presented to the immune system in complex with molecules of major histocompatibility complexes types I and II (Sartakova and Konenkov, 1997). Obviously, the differences in the representation of endogenous and exogenous antigens are important for the formation of protective immunity.

2.3.   Recombinant viruses

For the creation of live attenuated vaccines and inactivated vaccines, the search for attenuated strains of Dengue, West Nile virus, VEE, and Langathe continues. While previously weakened viruses were obtained through selection after long passages with high multiplicity of infection, the site-directed mutagenesis approach has recently become widespread. In this approach, nucleotide substitutions are introduced into cloned full-length DNA copies of flavivirus genomes using synthetic oligodeoxyribonucleotides (Maniatis et al., 1984), and subsequent *in vitro* transcription with phage RNA polymerases and RNA insertion into eukaryotic cells can lead to infectious attenuated viruses. Functionally important regions of the flavivirus genomes in which mutations lead to attenuation of pathogenic properties are the Z'-untranslated variant region (3'UTR), and sequences, encoding the cell receptor binding site, the glycosylation regions of prM, E, and NS1 proteins, fragments of the proteolytic cleavage of prM and NS1-NS2A proteins, and 8 C-terminal amino acid residues of the NS1 protein (Mandl et al., 1998). The most promising regions for modifications in the creation of live attenuated flavivirus vaccines are the non-coding regions of genomic RNA. Relatively large fragments of 3'-untranslated regions can be deleted from flavivirus genomes without losing infectivity. The reduced growth rate of such deletion mutants in cell cultures compared to the corresponding wild-type virus can very likely lead to a weakening of the pathogenic properties of the viruses. However, the absence of even small regions in the 5'-noncoding region and, especially, in the region of the long hairpin, results in non-viable mutants. Apparently, this is due to impaired interaction with cellular proteins, since deletion of the 82-87 n.o. fragment of Dengue virus RNA ensures selectivity of mutant reproduction towards host cells (Cahour et al., 1995). A similar feature of virus replication in phylogenetically different cell types was found for the vaccine strain 17D of yellow fever virus (Barrett et al., 1990).

Chimeric Dengue virus-based flaviviruses containing at least one or more structural genes of tick-borne or Japanese encephalitis viruses have been obtained (Pletnev et al., 1993). At the same time, point mutations or deletions were introduced into functionally important regions of the flavivirus genomes, resulting in weakened virulence (Pletnev et al., 1993).

Advances in genetic engineering allow the use of various attenuated DNA- and RNA-containing viruses as vectors for the expression of foreign genetic information (Hewson, 2000). Candidates for live vaccines against flavivirus infections can also be derived from recombinant smallpox virus expressing the surface glycoprotein E gene or NS3 protease gene (Khoretonenko et al., 2003; Konishi et al., 2008). Expression of E and M genes of Japanese encephalitis, yellow fever, and Dengue viruses cloned in recombinant poxviruses (smallpox, chickenpox, and canaries) leads to extracellular formation of subvirion particles inducing antibodies that inhibit erythrocyte hemagglutination and neutralize flaviviruses (Konishi *et al.*, 2008). It is possible to clone the complete coding sequence of flaviviruses into the genome of smallpox virus (Lai et al., 1991). Recombinant variola viruses expressing structural and some nonstructural VCE genes protect immunized mice from lethal infection (Dmitriev et al. , 1996). Currently, immunity against smallpox virus in vaccinated adults can lead to the elimination of recombinant smallpox virus-based viruses. However, the cessation of immunization of children with smallpox virus and the weakening of the immune response in the vaccinated population with age increases the prospects for the clinical use of recombinant vaccines based on this vector. A recombinant adenovirus expressing the VSE NS1 gene induces a humoral and cellular immune response and provides protection against lethal doses of the virus (Timofeev et al., 1998). Unfortunately, the immunomodulatory properties of many large DNA-containing viruses and the ability to integrate them into cellular genomes also limit their widespread use (Hewson, 2000). The advantages of RNA-containing viruses for creating recombinant vaccines are: 1) small genome sizes, typically 7,000 to 19,000 np, facilitating genetic engineering manipulations; 2) maturation of viruses in the cytoplasm of infected cells, providing high levels of expression of heterologous viral genes and eliminating the unpredictable effects of nuclear splicing of heterologous RNA 3) expression under the control of viral rather than cellular promoters eliminates complex multifactorial consequences; 4) the absence of DNA copies in the life cycle of such viruses results in the impossibility of integrating their genomes into the chromosomes of host cells; 5) short-term synthesis of viral proteins induces an immune response without danger of developing tolerance. Among viruses containing positive polarity genomic RNA, picornaviruses (in particular, poliovirus 2), alphaviruses (Semliki forest, Sindbis and Venezuelan equine encephalomyelitis viruses) and flaviviruses (Canjin virus) can be vectors for creating vaccines. Viruses containing negative polarity genomic RNA are also promising candidates, namely orthomyxoviruses (influenza virus), rhabdoviruses (vesicular stomatitis virus), and paramyxoviruses (measles virus) (Hewson, 2000). The expression system based on Semliki forest virus RNA has been developed and proven effective in immunizing mice against influenza viruses and Scottish sheep encephalomyelitis viruses. Thus, intraperitoneal injections of recombinant Semliki forest virus containing prM and E or NS1 genes of sheep Scots encephalomyelitis virus protected mice from infection with lethal doses of two different strains of this virus, while intranasal immunization resulted in a more limited protective effect (Fleeton et al., 1999). The obvious disadvantages of recombinant viruses are the expensive procedure of obtaining them in cell cultures and the impaired immune response due to the short-term simultaneous gene expression of several viruses (Liljeqvist and Stahl, 1999).

Unfortunately, the use of attenuated live vaccines is limited because of the possibility of reversion of the infectious agent to the wild type. Attenuation of RNA-containing viruses is particularly dangerous because of the variability of the genomes of such "quasispecies" in the absence of RNA repair systems in cells (Steinhauer and Holland, 1987; Martin et al., 2000). Extensive deletions of genome fragments of infectious agents could guarantee the safety of such vaccines, but their presence reduces the viability of mutants. Unfortunately, deletions of even short fragments of viral genomes are usually lethal (Cahour et al., 1995; Mandl et al., 1998). Only recombinant attenuated flaviviruses obtained by co-transfection of cell cultures with several plasmid DNAs with cloned genome fragments can ensure relative viral safety. Such approaches to vaccine creation are currently being developed by Safari Pasteur (USA). However, introduction of exogenous autoreplicons into dividing eukaryotic cells can lead to genetic rearrangements of both plasmids with disrupted structures of target viral genes and cellular genes or their regulatory elements (for references, see Morozova et al., 2000).

2.4.   Peptide and protein-based vaccines

Inactivated viruses, purified proteins and peptides are safer compared to live vaccines, but insufficiently effective. Inactivated vaccines are currently the most popular for the prevention of flavivirus infections (Mandl et al., 1989; Leonova, 2009). However, chemical inactivation of infectious agents can lead to partial disruption of the structure of antigenic determinants (Tsekhanovskaya et al., 1993). Disruption of infectivity of flaviviruses occurs as a result of partial denaturation of antigens during formaldehyde treatment or oxidation.

Exogenous antigens are introduced into the body several times in larger amounts than replicating attenuated viruses and exist in unchanged form for a relatively short time. At the same time, foreign proteins penetrate into cells, where they are broken down to peptides of 10 to 20 a.s. inside the endosomes during proteolytic processing (Sartakova and Konenkov, 1997). They then combine with major histocompatibility complex class II (MHC II) molecules to present complexes on the cell surface to CD4+-type T-helper lymphocytes (Th). Treatment of antigen-presenting cells with chloroquine, which inhibits hydrolysis of antigens within the endosomes, disrupts their binding to the major histocompatibility complex molecules. Antigens of inactivated viruses, recombinant proteins and their complexes in the form of virus-like particles, as well as various peptides are presented to the immune system only in complex with MHC II molecules (Sartakova and Konenkov, 1997). T helper proteins secrete interleukins 4 and 5 after vaccination, but not interferon- □ , which leads to a predominant humoral immune response and the synthesis of antibodies mainly of subclasses IgG1 and IgE (Tighea et al., 1998). The development of this humoral response contributes to the elimination of bacteria and extracellular virions. The absence of antigen-specific cytotoxic T lymphocytes (CD8+) prevents the elimination of intracellular viruses (Brower, 1998), and extracellular virions exist for a very short time. Inactivated vaccines require adjuvants and repeated immunizations, which increases their cost.

Recombinant proteins obtained in bacterial cells in the absence of posttranslational modification systems differ in the spatial structures of conformational epitopes from native antigens. In addition, recombinant proteins require a complex and expensive purification procedure. Such genetically engineered analogs have been described for all Flavivirus proteins, but despite their immunogenic properties, only the introduction of M, E, and NS1 proteins of the *Flavivirus* genus provides protection against infection. Patents have been issued for subunit vaccines consisting of recombinant proteins of Dengue and Japanese encephalitis flaviviruses. The C-terminal protein of the envelope of E virions is used to obtain its soluble form.

Eukaryotic heterologous viral gene expression systems including *Drosophila melanogaster* cells and yeast cells (Liljeqvist and Stahl, 1999) provide posttranslational modification and possibly proper protein stacking, but cultivation and purification methods are expensive.

Flavivirus antigens can form particles containing E and PrM or M proteins. Immunization of experimental animals with such virus-like particles provides a protective humoral immune response (Heinz et al., 1981). Unfortunately, the cost of obtaining and purifying virus-like particles consisting of the structural glycoproteins of flaviviruses is very high, so widespread use of such vaccines is not possible. Injections of individual purified VCE proteins caused the formation of specific antibodies that did not protect mice from infection (Pressman et al., 1993).

2.4.1 Anti-Diotypic Antigen Modeling Antibodies

Antidiotypic vaccines deserve special attention (Kullberg, 1978). The natural development of the immune response produces antibodies that react with the antigen and are themselves antigens for second antibodies. The second antibodies, also called anti-idiotic antibodies, can bind to different sites of the first antibodies. Some of the anti-idiotic antibodies that prevent the first antibodies from interacting with the antigen mimic the structure of the antigen and can be used as vaccines. Experimental anti-idiotypic vaccines against various infectious agents were obtained more than 30 years ago (Kullberg, 1978), but have not found practical application. Anti-idiotypic monoclonal antibodies secreted by hybrid cells and modeling epitopes of E VSE protein have been obtained and used for virological studies (Protopopova et al., 1996; 1997). Using such vaccines it is possible to induce an immune response to antigens not only of protein but also of polysaccharide nature. However, there is no information on the use of antidiotypic antibodies for the prevention of flavivirus infections. The high cost of work with eukaryotic cell cultures, the prohibition to introduce monoclonal antibodies secreted by mouse hybridomas to humans, and the danger of obtaining human hybrids serve as obstacles to the introduction of anti-idiotypic antibodies as vaccines.

2.4.2 Synthetic peptides

Synthetic linear peptides remain relatively weak immunogens even after conjugation with high-molecular-weight polymers (Volkova et al., 1998). For example, a linear synthetic peptide corresponding to the conserved 98 to 113 a.o.

protein E of VKE was conjugated to snail hemocyanin KLH, and virus neutralizing antibodies were detected as a result of immunization of rats (Volkova et al., 1998). In the free form, the linear peptides were nonimmunogenic, but after covalent attachment to KLH induced the formation of antibodies with high titers capable of neutralizing VKE with an index of 3.0 in immunized rats, whereas the neutralization index after immunization of rats with full-length glycoprotein E was 4.4 (Volkova et al., 1998).

Besides linear peptides corresponding to known B- (Tsekhanovskaya et al., 1993; Volkova et al., 1998) or T-cell epitopes of flaviviruses (Kutubuddin et al., 1991; Roehrig et al., 1992), in 1988 Tam proposed a new principle of creating conformational multiple antigenic peptides (MAPs) and direct synthesis of the peptide-antigen matrix by solid phase method (Tam, 1988). Multiple antigenic peptides or multipeptide antigens are synthetic macromolecules consisting of a matrix based on short peptides of trifunctional amino acid residues (usually 3 to 7 lysine amino acid residues), linked by peptide bonds and covalently attached to the amino groups of lysine residues of linear peptide antigens to form spatial macromolecules with

molecular weight up to 10 kDa (Fig. 14).

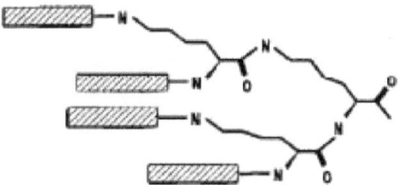

Figure 14: Structure of the tetravalent multiple antigenic peptide (MAP) based on the Lys-Lys-Lys tripeptide.

The undeniable advantages of MAPs are the high molar ratio and the dense packing of multiple copies of antigenic determinants, the possible combination of T-

and B-cell epitopes for a balanced immune response, and the absence of the screening effect of epitopes by nearby domains of high-molecular-weight proteins. Typically, the lysine core is less than 10% of the molecular weight of MAP. Despite the small size and molecular weight, MAP injections induce an immune response without conjugation of synthetic peptides with the carrier protein. In recent years, MAPs containing B- and/or T-cell epitopes of one or more antigens of various infectious agents have been used both for the induction of specific immune response and for diagnostic reactions (Nardin et al., 1995; Kruglov et al., 2009). At the same time, toxic properties, development of allergic reactions and other nonspecific effects for MAP, as well as for linear peptides, are still unknown.

Analysis of the variability of flavivirus proteins showed that one of the most conserved protein sites located on the virion surface is the fusion peptide. X-ray analysis of glycoprotein E revealed the presence of 3 domains I, II and III, as well as the presence of a "cd" loop at the top of domain II, which is the most conserved fragment of the E virion envelope protein, the "fusion peptide" (98113 a.s.), responsible for flavivirus entry into cells (for references see Seligman, 2008). In mature virions, a part of the fusion peptide of one of the monomers is under domains I and III of the neighboring monomer and is thus shielded from binding to antibodies to E protein. After receptor-mediated penetration of flaviviruses into the host cell endosomes, the partially hidden fusion peptide is released and E protein monomers form trimers (for references see Seligman, 2008). The partially surface localization and high conservativity of the fusion peptide among tick-borne flaviviruses make it promising for the development of new vaccines against tick-borne flaviviruses.

To induce a balanced humoral and cellular response, B- and T-cell epitopes must be included in synthetic peptide vaccines. B-cell epitopes of the virion envelope protein of flaviviruses are well known (Tsekhanovskaya et al., 1993). Epitope mapping of monoclonal antibodies to VCE protein E showed that viral neutralizing monoclonal antibodies have binding sites predominantly in the C-terminus of protein E with few exceptions (Tsekhanovskaya et al., 1993; Protopopova et al., 1996). However, the first attempts of immunization with synthetic peptides showed that a linear peptide corresponding to the conserved 98-113 a.s. of the N-terminal part of E protein of VSE and conjugated to snail hemocyanin (KLH) is capable of inducing virus-neutralizing antibodies (Volkova et al., 1998). Immunization of mice with synthetic peptides corresponding to the prM structural protein of Dengue flavivirus 2 and conjugated to bovine serum albumin (BSA) resulted in antibodies capable of neutralizing all 4 types of mosquito-borne Dengue flaviviruses (Vazquez et al., 2002).

To date, no single T-cell epitope of virion surface proteins conserved for all flaviviruses has been identified. Comparative analysis of the amino acid sequences of glycoprotein E of flaviviruses allowed the theoretical prediction of T helper binding sites based on the coincidence of the existence of amphiphilic segments, Rothbard-Taylor peptide and the predominantly alpha-helical secondary structure of the protein segment (Kutubuddin et al., 1991). A single cross-reactive T-cell epitope was predicted in the C-terminal portion (approximately 420-455 a. o.) of the E protein of all flaviviruses. Immunization of mice with synthetic peptides corresponding to the C-terminus of flaviviruses showed specific T cell proliferation (Kutubuddin et al., 1991). Analysis of T-cell epitopes for Dengue-2 and Murray Valley flaviviruses showed the greatest efficiency of cell proliferation *in vitro* and cytokine synthesis for a synthetic conserved peptide corresponding to 352-368 a. o. of Dengue-2 virus (Roehrig et al., 1992). The induction of antibodies by synthetic peptides including B-cell epitopes is stimulated when T-cell epitopes are added to the immunization mixture. The most effective immune response was observed with the introduction of covalently linked B- and T-cell epitopes in linear peptides (Roehrig et al., 1992).

Taking into account the data on the conserved structure of the "fusion peptide" of mite-borne flaviviruses, tetravalent multiple antigenic peptides (MAPs) containing fusion peptides and T-cell epitopes surrounded by short spacers and attached to a tripeptide of lysine amino acid residues were synthesized (Fig. 14). BALB/c mice were immunized intraperitoneally 4 times with 50-100 µg MAP. 7-10 days after the last immunization with 100 µg MAP in sera

The blood of immunized mice by enzyme immunoassay (ELISA) detected total antibodies to E protein of VEE with titers of 1:10,000 to 1:500,000 after immunization with FA4T5 MAP DRGWGNHCGLFGKGSIFTSLGKAVHQVFVKK (98 to 113 a.s. E protein of VEE, FT, 431 to 440 a.s. E protein of Dengue-4 virus (Kutubuddin et al, 1991), VKK) and 1:1.0001:100.000 postimmunizationFA4T4 DRGWGNHCGLFGKGSIGITVNPIVTEKDSPVNIEKK (98 - 113 a.o. protein E of VCE, G, 352 - 368 a.o. protein E of Dengue-2 virus (Roehrig et al., 1992). When the MAP dose was reduced to 50 µg, a decrease in ELISA titers of up to 1:1000 was observed. Reducing the time intervals between repeated immunizations to 10 days also resulted in a decrease in antibody titers to 1:1000. The obtained sera and ascites of mice contained specific polyclonal antibodies capable of binding to full-length glycoprotein E and recombinant truncated E protein, as well as with MAP FA4T4, FA4T5, and BFA linear peptide, and antibody titers in PIFA and ELISA with immobilized synthetic peptides were higher than those for immobilized full-length proteins (Table 5). Antibodies inhibiting hemagglutination of goose erythrocytes and virus-neutralizing antibodies were detected only after immunization with MAP FA4T5 containing 4 linear peptides DRGWGNHCGLFGKGSIFTSLGKAVHQVFVKK, attached to amino groups of matrix lysine residues (Table 5). Titers in RTGA for polyclonal antibodies after immunization of FA4T5 MAP mice ranged from 1:20 to 1:80 in different individuals depending on the time of blood sampling. Polyclonal antibodies from sera and ascites fluid of mice immunized with MAP FA4T5 neutralized 5 and 10 LD5o of tick-borne flaviviruses (VCE and Omsk hemorrhagic fever virus) at 1:2 dilution (Table 5), but did not neutralize 50 LD50 of different flaviviruses.

Table 5: Analysis of polyclonal antibodies after immunization of mice with MAP and monoclonal antibodies binding to flavivirus fusion peptide.

Antibody type	ELISA antibody titers for binding to E protein	ELISA antibody binding titers MAP	Titles RTGA	Plaque neutralization reaction titers on SPEV cell culture		Biological neutralization reaction titers in ICR mice	
				WCE	Powassan	WCE	OHL
Polyclonal antibodies of mice after immunization with MAP	1:1.000 1:100.000	1:1.000 1:100.000	-	-	-	-	-
Polyclonal antibodies of mice after immunization with MAP	1:10.000 1:500.000	1:10.000 1:500.000	1:20 1:80	1:8	1:64	1:2	1:2
MCA 10H10	1:50.000	1:100.000	1:640	-	1:64	-	-
MCA 1B1	1:10.000	-	1:320	1:128	-	1:4	1:4
MCA 10C2	1:100.000	1:50	1:40	-	-	-	-

Note: The "-" sign corresponds to negative reaction results.

Biological neutralization results are given for 10LD50 VKE and OHL.

The results of the neutralization of VCE and Povassan virus flaviviruses by polyclonal antibodies from mouse ascitic fluid immunized with MAP FA4T5 are shown in Fig. 15.

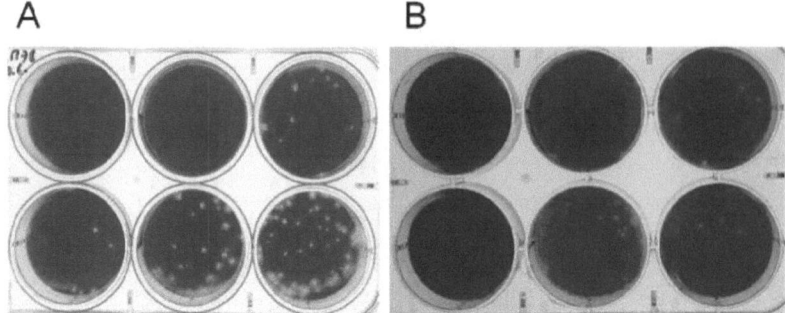

Figure 15: Results of neutralization of Powassan virus (A) and VCE (B) by polyclonal antibodies from mouse ascites fluid immunized with MAP FA4T5.

To evaluate the viral neutralizing and hemagglutination inhibitory properties, not only polyclonal antibodies after immunization of mice with MAP, but also monoclonal antibodies (MCA) obtained earlier (Matveev et al, 1989; Protopopova et al., 1996) and capable of binding to FA4T4 and FA4T5 MAPs as well as to a linear synthetic BFA peptide containing only flavivirus fusion peptide, as shown by PIFA and ELISA. A total of 6 MCAs, 1B1, 10C2, 10H10, 7F10, Fvn31, and Fvn32, were examined. Viral neutralizing properties were found for MCA 1B1 and 10H10 (Table 5).

Thus, MAPs were immunogenic in their free form, without conjugation to high-molecular-weight antigens. However, anti-hemagglutinins and viral neutralizing antibodies were detected only after immunization of FA4T5 MAP mice. Because the 16 N-terminal amino acid residues were the same in MAP FA4T4 and FA4T5, and induction of viral neutralizing and hemagglutination inhibiting antibodies was detected only after immunizing FA4T5 mice, the C-terminal amino acid residues of FA4T5 were more effective compared with FA4T4 because of the T cell epitope or spacers. Incorporation of the T-cell epitope SLGKAVHQVF into FA4T5 MAP resulted in the induction of antibodies that neutralized flaviviruses and inhibited hemagglutination. The optimal dose was 100 µg MAP to immunize one mouse, whereas previously 200 µg (in terms of peptide) of fusion peptide conjugate with KLH was used to immunize rats (Volkova et al., 1998) and 50 µg of linear peptides from prM protein in conjugate with BSA was used to effectively immunize mice (Vazquez et al., 2002).

The safety, low cost, chemical stability, ability to select conserved protein fragments with surface localization, high epitope density, antigenicity and immunogenicity of MAP allow the development of approaches to the prevention of various tick-borne RNA-containing flaviviruses as well as bacteria and protozoa.

Conclusion

Summarizing the results obtained, it is necessary to emphasize that when creating a new generation of vaccines against VEE, it is necessary to include nonstructural antigens and, especially, the NS1 glycoprotein in their composition. It is desirable to ensure the presentation of antigens to the immune system in association with the major histocompatibility complex type I to induce predominantly cellular protective immunity, since the presence of antibodies in blood and cerebrospinal fluid does not prevent the development of severe forms of tick-borne encephalitis. The combined use of safe inactivated or peptide vaccines in the initial stages of immunization followed by the use of RNA immunization or recombinant viruses with induction of predominantly cellular immune response through the Th-1 pathway and maintenance of lifelong immunity without the need for repeated injections is not excluded.

Acknowledgements

This work was partially supported by interdisciplinary grant No. 83 of the Siberian Branch of the Russian Academy of Sciences. In the section on the protective effect of the domestic vaccine Encevir in relation to Siberian strains of VEE, the data of Emma Anufrieva, which have not been published, were used. Unfortunately, Emma tragically died, but the authors always remember with gratitude and appreciation the years of joint work, emphasizing the deep erudition, diligence and extremely responsible attitude to work.

Bibliography

1. Avdeeva JI, Akolzina SE, Alpatova NA, Nikitina TN, Raschepkina MN, Medunitsyn NV. (2009) Effect of cytokines on the immunogenic properties of

the tick-borne encephalitis vaccine. Cytokines and inflammation. 2009. T. 8, № 2. http:ZZwww.cytokines.ru/2009/2ZArt2.php

2. Bergy (1980) A Brief Identifier of Bacteria, Mir, Moscow, 495 p.

3. Volkova TD, Volpina OM, Ivanova VT, Rubin SG, Semashko IV, Karavanov AS (1998) Study of the antigenic structure of tick-borne encephalitis virus using synthetic peptides. - Bioorganic Chemistry, Vol. 24, N2, pp. 100-111.

4. Vorobyeva M.S. (2002) Modern state of tick-borne encephalitis vaccine prophylaxis // In Book of tick-borne encephalitis. In: Vladivostok, 2002. C. 166-169.

5. Vorobyeva M.S. (2006) Tick-borne encephalitis. - Chapter in the collection "Do people need vaccines?" edited by Academician of RAMS Medunitsyn N.V., Moscow, 2006, pp. 134-141. 134-141.

6. Gendon, Y.Z. (1999) Viral mucosal vaccines. - Voprosy of Virology, Vol. 3, pp. 100-105.

7. Debabov V.G. (1997) DNA-vaccination and gene therapy based on transient expression of nucleic acids in human and animal somatic cells. - Molecular Biology, Vol. 31, N2, pp. 209-215.

8. Zlobin V.I., Mamaev L.V., Dzhioev Y.P., Kozlova I.V. (1996) Genetic types of tick-borne encephalitis virus. Journal of Infectious Pathology, Vol. 3, No. 4, pp. 13-17.

9. Zlobin V.I., Demina T.V., Belikov S.I. et al. (2001) Genetic typing of tick-borne encephalitis virus strains based on analysis of the homology of a fragment of the envelope protein gene. Voprosy of Virology, No 1, pp. 16-21.

10. Ignatiev G.M., Otrashevskaya E.V., Vorobyova M.S. (2003) Activity of cytokines during immunization with a vaccine against tick-borne encephalitis in experiment. Voprosy of Virology, No. 2, P. 22-25.

11. Karpenko L.I., Ignatiev G.M., Kozhina E.M., Kashentseva E.A., Poryvaeva V.A., Melamed N.V., Bayborodin S.I., Smirnova O.Yu., Illichev A.A. (2000) Production and study of recombinant strains of *Salmonella typhimurium* SL 7207, producing HBcAg and HBcAg-HBs. - Voprosy of Virology, N2, pp. 10-

14.

12. Korotkov Y.S., Nikitin A.N., Antonova A.M. (2007) Role. Climatic factors in the long-term dynamics of morbidity of the population of Irkutsk tick-borne encephalitis. Bulletin of All-Russian Scientific Center of the Siberian Branch of the Russian Academy of Medical Sciences, No.3 (55), p.121-125.

13. Kruglov I.V., Simonova T.V., Perez J.A., Haro I. (2009) Peculiarities of Antigen-antibody interactions using linear synthetic peptides and multipeptide antigen modeling antigenic determinants of hepatitis A virus. - Journal of Microbiology, Epidemiology and Immunology, No. 2. C. 31-34.

14. Kulberg A.Y. (1978) Anti-immunoglobulins. Antidiotypic antibodies. - Moscow, "Medicine", pp. 51-76.

15. Leonova G.N. (2009) Tick-borne encephalitis: current aspects. Moscow, Publisher I.V. Balabanov. 168 pp.

16. Lvov D.K., Klimenko S.M., Gaidamovich S.Y. (1989) Arboviruses and arbovirus infections. Moscow, "Medicine," 336 p.

17. Maniatis T., Fritsch E., Sambrook J. (1984) Molecular cloning. - Moscow, Mir, 480 p.

18. Matveev L.E., Karavanov A.S., Rubin S.G., Semashko I.V., Pressman E.K. (1989) Comparative evaluation of two immunoenzyme test systems for the detection of antibodies to tick-borne encephalitis virus. - Voprosy of Virology, Vol. 34, pp. 488-491.

19. Morozova O.V., Belyavskaya N.A., Matveev L.E., Kvetkova E.A., Pletnev A.G. (1990) Replicative complex of tick-borne encephalitis virus. II. Influence of envelope protein E and antibodies to it on RNA synthesis in vitro. - Bioorganic Chemistry, Vol. 16, No. 9, pp. 1277-1279.

20. Morozova O.V., Tkachev S.E., Chudinov A.R. (2006) RNA detection in the vaccine against tick-borne encephalitis Encevir. Voprosy of Virology, Vol. 51, No. 3, pp. 42-46.

21. Morozova O.V., Bakhvalova V.N. (2010) Natural cycles and tick-borne encephalitis. - "In the world of scientific discoveries," No. 2 Part 1, pp. 31-37.http://nkras.ru/issues.html http://nkras.ru/articles/2010/81/index.html.

22. Morozova O. V., Grishechkin A.E., Karan L.S., Isaeva E.I., Shchuchinova L.D., Loginova N.V., Zlobin V.I. (2011) Detection of tick-borne encephalitis virus in ixodid ticks collected in a natural focus of the Mountain Altai. Voprosy of virology, no. 2.

23. Pogodina V.V., Bochkova N.G., Koreshkova G.V. (1981) Properties of Aina/1448 serotype strains of tick-borne encephalitis virus. - Voprosy of Virology, N 6, C. 741-746.

24. Protopopova EV, Khusainova AD, Konovalova SN, Loktev VB. (1996) Preparation and study of the properties of anti-idiotypic antibodies carrying hemagglutinating paratopes of tick-borne encephalitis virus on their surface. - Voprosy of Virology, No.2, P.50-53.

25. Protopopova E.V., Konovalova S.N., Loktev V.B. (1997) Cell receptor isolation for tick-borne encephalitis virus using anti-idiotypic antibodies. - Voprosy of Virology, Vol. 42, No. 6, p. 264268.

26. Prokhorova O.G., Romanenko V.V., Zlobin V.I. (2006) Comparative Characteristics of the immunological activity of tick-borne encephalitis vaccines used in the mass vaccination campaign in the Sverdlovsk Region . Epidemiology and Vaccine Prophylaxis, Vol. 4(29), pp. 33-36.

27. Safronov P.F., Netesov S.V., Mikriukova T.P., Blinov V.M., Osipova

E.G., Kiseleva N.N., Sandakhcheev L.S. (1991) Nucleotide gene sequence and complete amino acid sequence of tick-borne encephalitis virus strain 205. Molecular Genetics, Microbiology and Virology, Vol. 4, pp. 23-29.

28. Sartakova M.L. and Konenkov V.I. (1997) Structural basis of intercellular interactions in the presentation of antigens to T-lymphocytes: histocompatibility complex molecules as one of the components of the trimolecular complex. - Adv. of modern biology. Vol. 117, issue 5, pp. 568-583.

29. Stronin OV, Surova Yu, Shutova NA, Shestakova AI, Sharova OI The effectiveness of vaccination against tick-borne encephalitis. Vestnik infektitologii i parazitologii ISSN 1609-9877, http://www.infectology.ru/publik/stat17. aspx.

30. Tsilinsky, J.J. (1988) Stability of species in RNA-genomic viruses. - The place of the species among biological systems. - Vilnius, P. 126-144.

31. Shapot V.S. (1968) Nucleases. - Moscow, "Medicine," 211 p.

32. Shchuchinova L.D. Epidemiological surveillance and control of tick-borne infections in the Altai Republic. D. thesis, 2009, Omsk.

33. Arguin P.M., Singleton J., Rotz L.D., Marston E., Treadwell T.A., Slater K., Chamberland M., Schwartz A., Tengelsen L., Olson J.G., Childs J.E. (1999) An investigation into the possibility of transmission of tick-borne pathogens via blood transfusion. Transfusion-Associated Tick-Borne Illness Task Force. Transfusion, V. 39(8), P. 828-833.

34. Bakhvalova V.N., Rar V.A., Tkachev S.E., Matveeva V.A., Matveev L.E., Karavanov A.S., Dobrotvorsky A.K. and Morozova O.V. (2000) Tick-borne encephalitis virus strains of Western Siberia. - Virus Research, V. 70 , № 1-2, P. 1-12.

35. Barrett A.D., Mathews J.H., Millen B.R., Ledger T.N., and Roehring J.T. (1990) Identification of monoclonal antibodies that distinguish between 17D 89

204 and other strains of yellow fever virus. - Journal of General Virology, V. 71, P. 13-18.

36. Bock H.L., Klockmann U., Jungst C., Schindel-Kunzel F., Theobald K., Zerban R. (1990) A new vaccine against tick-borne encephalitis: initial trial in man including a dose-response study. Vaccine, V. 8(1), P. 22-24.

37. Bot A., Bot S., Garcia-Sastre A. and Bona C. (1996) DNA immunization of newborn mice with a plasmid-expressing nucleoprotein of influenza virus. - Viral Immunology, V. 9, N4, P. 207-210.

38. Brower V. (1998) Naked DNA vaccines come of age. - Nature Biotechnology, V. 16, P. 1304-1305.

39. Cahour A., Pletnev A., Vazeille-Falcoz M., Rosen L. and Lai C.-J. (1995) Growth-restricted Dengue virus mutants containing deletions in the 5' noncoding region of the RNA genome. - Virology, V. 207, P. 1-9.

40. Carr J.P. and Zaitlin M. (1993) Replicase-mediated resistance. - Seminars in Virology, V. 4, P. 339-347.

41. Chen H.W., Pan C.H., Liau M.Y., Jou R., Tsai C.J., Wu H.J., Lin Y.L., Tao M.H. (1999) Screening of protective antigens of Japanese encephalitis virus by DNA immunization: a comparative study with conventional viral vaccines. - Journal of Virology, V. 73, N12, P. 10137-10145.

42. Chin J., Turner B., Barchia I. And Mullbacher A. (2000) Immune response to orally consumed antigens and probiotic bacteria. - Imminology and Cell Biology, V. 78, P. 55-66.

43. Cohen J. (1993) Naked DNA points way to vaccines. - Science, V. 259, P. 1691-1692.

44. Corthesy-Theulaz I.E., Hopkins S., Bachmann D., Saldinger P.F., Porta N., Haas R., Zheng-Xin Y., Mayer T., Blum A.L., Kraehenbuhl J.-P. (1998) Mice are protected from *Helicobacter pylori* infection by nasal immunization with attenuated *Salmonella typhimurium* [phoPc] expressing urease A and B subunits. - Infect. Immunol., V. 66, P. 581-586.

45. Dmitriev I.P., Khromykh A.A., Ignatyev G.M., Gainullina M.N., Ageenko

V.A., Dryga S.A., Vorobyeva M.S., Sandakhchiev L.S. (1996) Immunization with recombinant vaccinia viruses expressing structural and part of the nonstructural region of tick-borne encephalitis virus cDNA protect mice against lethal encephalitis. - J. Biotechnol. , V. 44, N1-3, P. 97-103.

46. Dowty M.E., Williams P., Zhang G. (1995) Plasmid DNA entry into postmitotic nuclei of primary rat myotubes. - Proc. Natl. Acad. Sci. USA, V. 92, P. 4572-4576.

47. Ecker M., Allison S.L., Meixner T., Heinz F.X. (1999) Sequence analysis and genetic classification of tick-borne encephalitis viruses from Europe and Asia. - Journal of General Virology, V. 80, P. 179-185.

48. Finn G.K., Kurz B.W., Cheng R.Z., Shmookler R.J. (1989) Homologous plasmid recombination is elevated in immortally transformed cells. - Mol. Cell. Biol. , V. 9, P. 4009-4017.

49. Fleeton M.N., Sheahan B.J., Gould E.A., Atkins G.J., Liljestrom P. (1999) Recombinant Semliki Forest virus particles encoding the prME or NS1 proteins of louping ill virus protect mice from lethal challenge. - Journal of General Virology, V. 80, P. 1189-1198.

50. Heinz F.X., Tuma W., Kunz C. (1981) Antigenic and immunogenic properties of defined physical forms of TBEV structural proteins. - Infectious Immunology, V. 33, N1, P.250-257.

51. Heinz F.X. and Mandl C.W. (1993) The molecular biology of tick-borne encephalitis virus. - Apmis, N101, P. 735-745.

52. Heinz F.X., Holzmann H., Essl A., Kundi M. (2007) Field effectiveness of vaccination against tick-borne encephalitis. - Vaccine. V. 25(43), P. 75597567.

53. Hewson R. A. (2000) RNA viruses: emerging vectors for vaccination and gene therapy. - Molecular Medicine Today, V.6, P. 28-35.

54. Hofmann H. (1973) The nonspecific defense in neurotropic arbovirus infections. Zbl. Bakt. Hyg. I. Dept. Orig. A223, P.143-163.

55. Hosie M.J., Flynn J.N., Rigby M.A., Cannon C., Dunsford T., Mackay N.A., Argyle D., Willett B.J., Miyazawa T., Onions D.E., Jarrett O. and Neil J.C. (1998) DNA vaccination affords significant protection against feline immunodeficiency virus infection without inducing detectable antiviral antibodies. - Journal of Virology, V. 72, N9, P. 7310-7319.

5 6. Ilyin Y.V. and Georgiev G.P. (1982) The main types of organization of genetic material in eukaryotes. - CRC Crit. Rev. Biochem., V. 12, P. 237.

57. Jurka J. and Smith T. (1988) A fundamental division in the Alu family of repeated sequences. - Proc. Natl. Acad. Sci. USA, V. 85, P. 4775-4778.

58. Karlin S., Doerfler W. and Cardon L.R. (1994) Why is CpG suppressed in the genomes of virtually all small eukaryotic viruses but not in those of large eukaryotic viruses? - Journal of Virology, V.68, N5, P.2889-2897.

59. Khoretonenko M.V., Vorovitch M.F., Zakharova L.G., Pashvykina G.V., Ovsyannikova N.V., Stephenson J.R., Timofeev A.V., Altstein A.D., Shneider A.M. (2003) Vaccinia virus recombinant expressing gene of tick-borne encephalitis virus non-structural NS1 protein elicits protective activity in mice. - Immunology Letters, V.90, N2-3, P. 161-163; Erratum in: Immunology Letters, 2004 V.91, N2-3, P.255.

60. Konishi E., Yagawa K., Yamanaka A. (2008) Vero cells infected with vaccinia viruses expressing Japanese encephalitis virus envelope protein induce polykaryocyte formation under neutral conditions. J Infect Dis. V. 61, N5, P. 410-411.

61. Krieg A.M., Gmelig-Meyling F., Gourley M.F., Kisch W.J., Chrisey L.A. and Steinberg A.D. (1991) Uptake of oligodeoxyribonucleotides by lymphoid cells is heterogeneous and inducible. - Antisense Research and Development, V. 1, P. 161-171.

62. Kutubuddin M., Kolaskar A.S., Galande S., Gore M.M., Ghosh S.N., Banerjee K. (1991) Recognition of helper T cell epitopes in envelope (E) glycoprotein of Japanese encephalitis, west Nile and Dengue viruses. - Mol Immunol. , V. 28, N1-2, P. 149-154.

63. Lai C.-J., Zhao B., Hori H., Bray M. (1991) Infectious RNA transcribed from stably cloned full-length cDNA of dengue type-4 virus. - Proc. Natl. Acad. Sci. USA, V. 88, P. 5139-5143.

64. Leclerc C., Martineau P., van der Werf S., Deriaud E., Duplay P., Hofnung M. (1990) Induction of virus-neutralizing antibodies by bacteria expressing the C3 poliovirus epitope in the periplasm. The route of immunization influences the isotypic distribution and the biological activity of the antipoliovirus antibodies. - J. Immunol., V. 144, P. 3174-3182.

65. Liljeqvist S. and Stahl S. (1999) Production of recombinant subunit vaccines: protein immunogens, live delivery systems and nucleic acid vaccines. - Journal of Biotechnology, V. 73, P. 1-33.

66. Lin Y.L., Chen L.K., Liao C.L., Yeh C.T., Ma S.H., Chen J.L., Huang Y.L., Chen S.S., Chiang H.Y. (1998) DNA immunization with Japanese encephalitis virus nonstructural protein NS1 elicits protective immunity in mice. - Journal of Virology, V. 72, N1, P. 191-200.

67. Locht C. (2000) Live bacterial vectors for intranasal delivery of protective antigens. - Pharmaceutical Science and Technology Today, V. 3, P. 121-128.

68. Loke S.L., Stein C.A., Zhang X.H., Mori K., Nakanishi N., Subasinghe S., Cohen J.S. and Neckers L.M. (1989) Characterization of oligonucleotide transport into living cells. - Proc. Natl. Acad. Sci. USA, V. 86, P. 3474-3478.

69. MacGregor G.R., James M.R., Arlett C.F., Burke J.F. (1987) Analysis of mutations occurring during replication of SV-40 shuttle vector in mammlian cells. - Mutat. Res., V. 183, P. 273-278.

70. Mandl C.W., Heinz F.X., Stockl E. and Kunz C. (1989) Genome sequence of tick-borne encephalitis virus (Western sybtype) and comparative analysis of nonstructural proteins with other flaviviruses. - Virology, V. 173, N1, P. - 291301.

71. Mandl C.W., Holzmann H., Meixner T., Rauscher S., Stadler P.F., Allison S.L. and Heinz F.X. (1998) Spontaneous and engineered deletions in the 3' noncoding region of tick-borne encephalitis virus: construction of highly

attenuated mutants of a flavivirus. - Journal of Virology, V. 72, №3, P. - 21322140.

72. Mansfield K.L., Johnson N., Phipps L.P., Stephenson J.R., Fooks A.R., Solomon T. (2009) Tick-borne encephalitis virus - a review of an emerging zoonosis. J. Gen. Virol. 90(Pt 8), P. 1781-1794.

73. Marth E. and Kleinhappl B. (2002) Albumin is necessary stabilizer of TBE vaccine to avoid fever in chidren after vaccination. - Vaccine, N20, P. 532537.

74. Martin J., Ferguson G.L., Wood D.J., Minor P.D. (2000) The vaccine origin of the 1968 epidemic of type 3 poliomyelitis in Poland. Virology. V. 278, N1, P. 42-49.

75. Martinez X., Brandt C., Saddallah F., Tougne C., Barrios C., Wild F., Dougan G., Lambert P.-H., and Siegrist C.-A. (1997) DNA immunization circumvents deficient induction of T helper type 1 and cytotoxic T lymphocyte responses in neonates and during early life. - Proc. Natl. Acad. Sci. USA, V. 94, P. - 87268731.

76. Mathew A., Kurane I., Rothman A.L., Zeng L.L., Brinton M.A., Ennis F.A. (1996) Dominant recognition by human CD8+ cytotoxic T lymphocytes of dengue virus nonstructural proteins NS3 and NS 1.2a. - Journal of Clinical Investigations, V. 98, N7, P. 1684-1691.

77. Matveeva V.A., Popova R.V., Kvetkova E.A., Chernicina L.O., Zlobin V.I., Puchovskaya N.M., Morozova O.V. (1995) Antibodies against tick-borne encephalitis virus (TBEV) non-structural and structural proteins in human sera and spinal fluid. - Immunology Letters, V. 46, N1-2, P. 1-4.

78. Mayer V., Ernek E., Blaskovic D., Kozuch O., Nosek J. (1967) Study on the virulence of tick-borne encephalitis virus. VII. Immunogenicity of attenuated virus (clone HY-HK 28 "28") for goats, cattle and sheep. Acta Virol., V.11, P. 334-345.

79. Mayer V. (1973) Humoral antibody response in volunteers given the live, highly attenuated "14" clone derived from Langat E5 virus. Acta Virol. V.17, P. 367.

80. Monath T.P. (1986) Pathobiology of the flaviviruses. Plenum Press, New York-London, P. 375-440.

81. Moreau J., Marcaud L., Maschat F., Kejzlarova-Lepesant J., Lepesant J.A. and Scherrer K. (1982) A+T-rich linkers define functional domains in eukaryotic DNA. - Nature, V. 295, P. 260-262.

82. Morozova O. V., Maksimova T.G., Kostenko E.V. (2000) EBV-based plasmid DNA rearrangements after transfection of eukaryotic cells. - Plasmid. V. 43, N3, P.185-189.

83. Nakai D., Seita T., Terasaki T. (1996) Cellular uptake mechanism for oligonucleotides: involvement of endocytosis in the uptake of phosphodiester oligonucleotides by a human colorectel adenocarcinoma cell line, HCT-15. - Jouranl of Pharmacology and Experimental Therapy, V. 278, P. 1362-1372.

84. Nardin E.H., Oliveira G.A., Calvo-Calle J.M., Nussenzweig R.S. (1995) The use of MAPs in the analysis and induction of protective immune responses against infectious diseases. - Adv. Immunol., V. 60, P. 105-149.

85. Nguyen T.N., Gourdon M.-H., Hansson M., Robert A., Samuelson P., Libon C., Andreoni C., Nygren P.-A., Binz H., Uhlen M., Stahl S. (1995) Hydrophobicity engineering to facilitate surface display of heterologous gene products on *Staphylococcus xylosus*. - J. Biotechnol., V. 42, P. 207-219.

86. Nichols W.W., Ledwith B.J., Manam S.V., Troilo P.J. (1995) Potential DNA vaccine integration into host cell genome. - Ann. NY Acad. Sci., V. 772, P. - 3039.

8 7. O'Sullivan D.J. and Klaenhammer T.R. (1993) High- and low-copy-number Lactococcus shuttle cloning vectors with features for clone screening. - Gene, V. 137, N2, P. 227-231.

88. Palukaitis P. and Zaitlin M. (1997) Replicase-mediated resistance to plant virus disease. - Adv. Vir. Res., V. 48, P. 349-377.

89. Peiris J.S.M. and Porterfield J.S. (1979) Antibody-mediated enhancement of flavivirus replication in macrophage cell lines. - Nature (London), V. 282, P. 509.

90. Phillpotts R.J., Stephenson J.R., Porterfield J.S. (1985) Antibody-dependent enhancement of tick-borne encephalitis virus infectivity. - Journal of General Virology, V. 66, N8, P. 1831-1837.

91. Phillpotts R.J., Venugopal K., Brooks T. (1996) Immunization with DNA polynucleotides protects mice against lethal challenge with St. Louis encephalitis virus. - Archives of Virology, V. 141, N3-4, P. 743-749.

92. Plassmann E. (1980) Tick-borne encephalitis also from infected milk. Arztl. Praxis, v. 32. p. 2025-2026.

93. Pletnev A.G., Yamshchikov V.F., Blinov V.M. (1990) Nucleotide sequence of the genome and complete amino acid sequence of the polyprotein of TBE. - Virology, V. 174, P. 250-263.

94. Pletnev A.G., Bray M., Lai C.J. (1993) Chimeric tick-borne encephalitis and dengue type 4 viruses: effects of mutations on neurovirulence in mice. - J. Virol. V. 67, N8, P.4956-4963.

95. Pouwels P.H., Leer R.J., Boersma W.J. (1996) The potential of Lactobacillus as a carrier for oral immunization: development and preliminary characterization of vector systems for targeted delivery of antigens. - Journal of Biotechnology, V. 44, N1-3, P. 183-192.

96. Powell S., Whitaker S., Peacock J., and Mcmillan T. (1993) Ataxia telangiectasia: an investigation of the repair defect in cell line AT5BIVA by plasmid reconstitution. - Mutat. Res., V. 294, P. 9-20.

97. Pressman E.K., Karavanov A.S., Matveeva V.A., Matveev L.E., Pugachev K.V. and Vinogradova I.V. (1993) Comparative analysis of serological activity of non-structural protein (NS1) from tick-borne encephalitis virus and its analog expressed in bacterial cells. - Immunology Letters, V. 38, P. 173-178.

98. Raz E., Carson D.A., Parker S.E., Parr T.B., Abai A.M. , Aichinger G., Gromkowski S.H., Singh M., Lew D., Yankauckas M.A., Baird S.M. and Rhodes G.H. (1994) Intradermal gene immunization: The possible role of

DNA uptake in the induction of cellular immunity to viruses. Proc. Natl. Acad. Sci. USA, V. 91, P. 9519-9523.

99. Rodriguez F., An L.L., Harkins S., Zhang J., Yokoyama M., Widera G., Fuller

J .T., Kincaid C., Campbell I.L. and Whitton J.L. (1998) DNA immunization with minigenes: low frequency of memory cytotoxic T lymphocytes and inefficient antiviral protection are rectified by ubiquitination. - Journal of Virology, V. 72, N6, P. 5174-5181.

100.   Roehrig J.T., Johnson A.J., Hunt A.R., Beaty B.J., Mathews J.H. (1992) Enhancement of the antibody response to flavivirus B-cell epitopes by using homologous or heterologous T-cell epitopes. - J Virol., V. 66, N6, P. - 33853390.

101.   Schlesinger J.J., Brandriss M.W., Walsh E.E. (1985) Protection against 17D yellow fever encephalitis in mice by passive transfer of monoclonal antibodies to the nonstructural glycoprotein gp48 and by active immunization with gp48. - Journal of Immunology, V. 135, N4, P. 2805-2809.

102.   Schmaljohn C., Vanderzanden L., Bray M., Custer D., Meyer B., Li D., Rossi C., Fuller D., Fuller J., Haynes J., Huggins J. (1997) Naked DNA vaccines expressing the prM and E genes of Russian spring summer encephalitis virus and Central European encephalitis virus protect mice from homologous and heterologous challenge. - Journal of Virology, V. 71, N12, P. 9563-9569.

103.   Schwartz R.S. (1988) Polyvalent anti-DNA autoantibodies: immunochemical and biological significance. - Int. Rev. Immunol., V. 3, P. 97-115.

104.   Seligman S.J. (2008) Constancy and diversity in the flavivirus fusion peptide. - Virol. J.,V. 5, P. 27-37.

105.   Sheets R, Petricciani J. (2004) Vaccine cell substrates 2004. Expert Rev Vaccines. V. 3(6), P. 633-638.

106.   Smorodintsev A., Dubov A., Ilyenko V., Platonov V (1969) A new

approach to development of live vaccine against tick-borne encephalitis. J. Hyg., V. 67, P. 13-20.

107.   Sparwasser T., Miethke T., Lipford G., Erdmann A., Hacker H., Heeg K ., Wagner H. (1997) Macrophages sense pathogens via DNA motifs: induction of tumor necrosis factor D-mediated shock. - European Journal of Immunology, V. 27, N7, P. 1671-1679.

108.   Stephenson J.R., Lee J.M., Bailey N., Shepherd A.G., Melling J. (1991) Adjuvant effect of human growth hormone with an inactivated flavivirus vaccine. J Infect Dis. , V. 164(1), P. 188-191.

109.   Steinhauer A. and Holland J.J. (1987) Rapid evolution of RNA viruses. - Annual Review of Microbiology, V. 41, P. 409-433.

110.   Sundaram P., Xiao W., Brandsma J.L. (1996) Particle-mediated delivery of recombinant expression vectors to rabbit skin induces high-titered polyclonal antisera (and circumvents purification of a protein immunogen). - Nucleic Acids Research, V. 24, N7, P. 1375-1377.

111.   Tam J. P. (1988) Synthetic peptide vaccine design: synthesis and properties of a high-density multiple antigenic peptide system. - Proc. Natl. Acad. Sci. U S A, V. 85, N15, P. 5409-5413.

112.   Tang D., DeVit M., Johnston S.A. (1992) Genetic immunization is a simple method for eliciting an immune response. - Nature, V. 356, P. 152-154.

113.   Taubes G. (1997) Salvation in a snippet of DNA? - Science, V. 278, P. 1711-1714.

114.   Thomas D.B. (1993) Viruses and the cellular immune response. - New York, Basel, Hong Kong.

115.   Tick-Borne Encephalitis (TBE) and its Immunoprophylaxis. Immuno AG, Vienna, Austria, 1996.

116.   Tighea H., Corra M., Romanb M. and Raz E. (1998) Gene vaccination: plasmid DNA is more than just a blueprint. - Immunology Today, V. 19, P. - 8997.

117.   Timofeev A.V., Ozherelkov S.V., Pronin A.V., Deeva A.V., Karganova G.G., Elbert L.B. and Stephenson J.R. (1998) Immunological basis for protection in a murine model of tick-borne encephalitis by a recombinant adenovirus carrying the gene encoding the NS1 non-structural protein. - Journal of General Virology, V. 79, P. 689-695.

118.   Timofeev A.V., Karganova G.G. (2003) Tick-borne enecephalitis vaccine: from past to future. Moscow, Pronto Prints, Ltd, 44 pp.

119.   Tsekhanovskaya N.A., Matveev L.E., Rubin S.G., Karavanov A.S. and Pressman E.K. (1993) Epitope analysis of tick-borne encephalitis (TBE) complex viruses using monoclonal antibodies to envelope glycoprotein of TBE virus (persulcatus subtype). - Virus Research, V. 30, P. 1-16.

120.   Vazquez S, Guzman MG, Guillen G, Chinea G, Perez AB, Pupo M, Rodriguez R, Reyes O, Garay HE, Delgado I, Garcia G, Alvarez M. (2002) Immune response to synthetic peptides of dengue prM protein. - Vaccine, V. 20, no. 13-14, P. 1823-1830.

121.   Vlassov V.V., Yakubov L.A., Karamyshev V., Pautova L., Rykova E., and Nechaeva M. (1995) In vivo pharmacokinetics of oligonucleotides following administration by different routes. In: Delivery strategies for antisense oligonucleotide therapeutics. Akhtar S. (Ed.), CRC Press, P. 71-83.

122.   WHO Cell culture as a substrate for the production of influenza vaccine: memorandum from a WHO meeting. (1995) Bull. Wld Hlth Org., V. 73, P. 431 - 435.

123.   Winegar R.A., Monforte J.A., Suing K.D. (1996) Determination of tissue distribution of an intramuscular plasmid vaccine using PCR and in situ DNA hybridization. - Hum. Gene Ther., V. 7, P. 2185-2194.

124.   Wolff J.A., Malone R.W., Williams P. (1990) Direct gene transfer into mouse muscle in vivo. - Science, V. 247, P. 1465-1468.

125.   Wolff J.A., Dowty M.E., Jiao S. (1992) Expression of naked plasmids by cultured myotubes and entry of plasmids into T tubules and caveolae of mammalian sceletal muscle. - Journal of Cellular Science, V. 103, P. 1249 -

1259.

126. Xiang R., Lode H.N., Chao T.H., Ruehlmann J.M., Dolman C.S., Rodriguez F., Whitton J.L., Overwijk W.W., Restifo N.P., Reisfeld R.A. (2000) An autologous oral DNA vaccine protects against murine melanoma. Proc Natl Acad Sci U S A, V. 97(10), P. 5492-5497.

127. Xiong S., Gerloni M., Zanetti M. (1997) In vivo role of B lymphocytes in somatic transgene immunization. - Proc. Natl. Acad. Sci. USA, V. 94, P. 6352-6357.

128. Yakubov L.A., Deeva E.A., Zarytova V.F., Vlassov V.V. (1989) Mechanism of oligonucleotide uptake by cells: involvement of specific receptors? - Proc. Natl. Acad. Sci. USA, V.86, P. 6454-6458.

129. Yates J.L., Warren N., Sugden B. (1985) Stable replication of plasmid derived from Epstein-Barr virus in various mammalian cells. - Nature, V. 313, P. 812-815.

130. Zhu N., Liggitt T., Liu Y., Debs R. (1993) Systemic gene expression after intravenous DNA delivery into adult mice. - Science, V.261, P. 209-211.

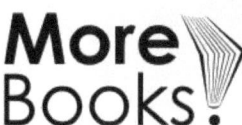
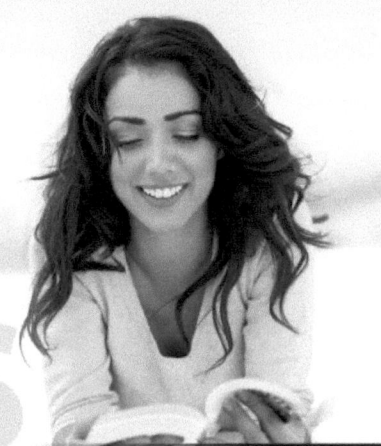

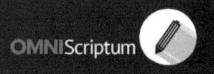

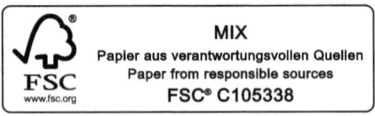